The Swift Diet

The Swift Diet

4 Weeks to

Mend the Belly, Lose the Weight, and Get Rid of the Bloat

KATHIE MADONNA SWIFT, MS, RDN
and JOSEPH HOOPER

Foreword by **MARK HYMAN, MD**

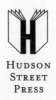

HUDSON
STREET
PRESS

HUDSON STREET PRESS
Published by the Penguin Group
Penguin Group (USA) LLC
375 Hudson Street
New York, New York 10014

USA | Canada | UK | Ireland | Australia | New Zealand | India | South Africa | China
penguin.com
A Penguin Random House Company

First published by Hudson Street Press, a member of Penguin Group (USA) LLC, 2014

REGISTERED TRADEMARK—MARCA REGISTRADA

HUDSON
STREET
PRESS

ISBN 978-1-59463-332-4

Printed in the United States of America
1   3   5   7   9   10   8   6   4   2

Set in Minion Pro with News Gothic MT Std and Bell MT
Designed by Daniel Lagin

To my sweet granddaughters, Lauren and Sydney,
who have been blessed with a healthy start, and to your delicious
journey through a nourishing life. And to all our little ones,
who deserve the very best food served with love.

CONTENTS

FOREWORD

Ten years ago, Kathie Swift, our nurse partner Nina Silver and I holed up in my red-shingled house in western Massachusetts and together became the UltraWellness Center. For those first few months, I was working in my office upstairs, Nina was in the living room and Kathie, as befitting my head of nutrition, was in the dining room, just off the kitchen. Today, the functional medicine center that Kathie, Nina and I built employs a staff of thirty working out of a well-equipped building set against the Berkshires woods. Kathie, of course, played an important role in that growth and success. In fact it was she who first pointed me toward what we now call functional medicine, an approach that seeks to uncover the root causes of disease, always with the emphasis on healthy diet and lifestyle.

When we were both working at the Canyon Ranch spa in the Berkshires in the nineties, Kathie introduced cutting-edge nutritional medicine concepts to the doctors and nutritionists there. And she introduced me to Dr. Jeffrey Bland, the father of functional medicine, who became a mentor to so many of us. At Canyon Ranch, where I was co–medical director and Kathie the nutrition director, we were able develop and apply these functional medicine ideas in a clinical setting. Although I was that rare doctor who had actually studied nutrition in a serious way, it was Kathie who really taught me to think rigorously about the role of nutrition in health. In contrast to the "pill for every ill" mentality that almost every doctor absorbs in medical training, with Kathie's help I came to see how food itself could be powerful medicine with which to treat and actually reverse disease. She was so open and enthusiastic about partnering with me at the Ranch, and together we refined an approach that was effective for thousands of clients there. When I left Canyon Ranch, to build the UltraWellness Center, she was the first person I called to join me. Since then, she's helped me with several of my books, including *UltraMetabolism*, to which she contributed the recipes. (As you'll see in *The Swift Diet*, Kathie is an accomplished and creative home cook.)

It's no accident that Kathie and I share this quest to push beyond conventional medical wisdom. We both had to figure out how to heal ourselves before we could fully help our patients. I've written about my struggle with chronic fatigue and mercury poisoning in a number of my books. Here in *The Swift Diet*, Kathie opens up for the first time about her battle with chronic fatigue syndrome brought on by an undiagnosed sensitivity to gluten. Her success in healing herself with a high-fiber, mostly plant-based diet fuels her passion to find the right answers for clients and readers with gut and weight issues. And she never stops. She has the ability to synthesize enormous amounts of data in order to connect the dots, to create meaning where there was none. In *The Swift Diet* she draws on the latest research on the role of gut bacteria to distill a practical step-by-step guide to health and healthy weight loss.

I think the microbiome is an enormously important emerging story. We're seeing that the bacteria that live in the gut help regulate the interlocking systems in the body, including the immune system and insulin metabolism. I've seen it in the research literature and I've seen it in clinical practice: different diets can have different effects on weight, even though they may contain the same number of calories, because of how they affect the gut bacteria. Kathie has been at the forefront of this field, giving talks around the country to general audiences and to her professional peers. She's been the driving force behind the Dietitians in Integrative and Functional Medicine within the Academy of Nutrition and Dietetics, she's a founding member of the Institute for Functional Medicine's nutrition advisory board and, for the past decade, she's organized an influential annual conference on health and nutrition, Food As Medicine, sponsored by the Center for Mind-Body Medicine in Washington, DC, where I've been honored to serve on the faculty and board of directors. Kathie has become something close to a one-woman bridge between the worlds of functional medicine and mainstream nutrition.

She's also adept at making the connection between body and spirit. Over the past seven years, as she's developed and led workshops on weight loss, digestion and detox at the Kripalu Center in the Berkshires, she's integrated mind-body techniques into her nutrition work, addressing the stress piece of the health and weight-loss puzzle. Just as I started out my career as a yoga instructor, Kathie is now a certified qigong teacher!

My friend and colleague Kathie Swift is one of the leading innovators in nutrition in this country. She has devoted her life to discovering how we can heal ourselves through food, and she's inspired a host of others to do the same. If you've bought *The Swift Diet*, you're about to join that select but growing group.

—Mark Hyman, MD

The Swift Diet

Chapter 1

SCIENCE, WISDOM AND STORY

SELF-INQUIRY BOX

1. Have you noticed that when you're having digestive problems, it's difficult to manage your weight? That there is a connection between "Irritable Bowel" and "Irritable Weight"?
2. Have you noticed that a week of high stress can have a similar effect on your belly as a course of antibiotics? That both can seem to throw your entire digestive system off?
3. Have you noticed that when you're eating more vegetables and fruits, and less meat and processed foods, you feel lighter and more energetic?

If you've picked up this book, there's an excellent chance that you're frustrated with your weight. Maybe you're carrying around an extra ten or twenty or fifty pounds that you can't seem to keep off. Odds are you've gone on diets before and you may have had success, for a while, but you couldn't handle the feeling of deprivation, of being hungry over the long haul, and the unwanted weight came back. Or the diet was one of those complicated multiphase productions and after a while you lost the patience or the will to precisely track your calorie intake or the ratio of carbs/fats/protein you were supposed to be eating in any given week.

But there's an easier and a better way. It happens to be supported by what has become very possibly the most significant and compelling scientific story to unfold in this century—the impact of the bacteria that live in our gut on most every facet of our lives: our weight, our digestive health, our immune system response, our *emotions*, virtually every aspect of our being. For instance, these gut bacteria can produce toxins that leak into the bloodstream, creating a system-wide inflammation that pushes the body to store calories as fat rather than burning them as energy, *and* it can drive food cravings. (Researchers now recognize this "metabolic endotoxemia," literally a poisoning from within, as a likely under-the-radar driver of obesity in this country.) Amazingly, these same bacteria can influence the production of gut hormones that speak directly to the brain, signaling either fullness or hunger. The good news is that by paying attention to what you eat and how you live—chronic stress causes major dysfunction in the gut— you can exert control over the process. Take care of your gut bacteria and they'll take care of you!

But we're getting ahead of ourselves. Let's return to weight gain, which for many women is the most distressing sign that all is not right with the belly and the body.

The Belly Blues

The weight of the average American woman has gone up twenty pounds since the early seventies. Today, 33 percent of American adults are considered overweight (a body mass index of 25 to 30) and 35 percent obese (a BMI over 30). Over the past twenty years, the obese group has increased in number by 60 percent, giving us a new label, the "obesity epidemic," and fears about crushing rates of heart disease and type 2 diabetes in the future. What hasn't been talked about as much is that during this same period of time, the nation has experienced a second epidemic, one that has been taking place, out of sight, but not out of mind, in the bellies of American women.

Consider: While men and women have suffered that weight gain in roughly equal measure, women are twice as likely as men to have the chronic, low-grade digestive complaints that get lumped together as irritable bowel syndrome, affecting an estimated 30 percent of American women. Digestive problems are compounded by food allergies and sensitivities, especially to the family of proteins found in gluten-containing grains like wheat, rye and barley. Conservatively estimated, 1 percent of the American population is afflicted with celiac disease, a severe intolerance to gluten. Six times that number have a less severe sensitivity to gluten, which can still result in serious digestive problems as well as all-over fatigue and depression. (Again, a conservative estimate. I, and many nutritionists, find that *many* of our female clients feel better without gluten.) And it doesn't stop there. Clinical evidence is piling up that huge swaths of the population are suffering from gut-disturbing, and likely weight-frustrating, sensitivities to common dietary elements like lactose in dairy products, fructose in high-fructose corn syrup and related compounds found in some legumes and vegetables.

The belly of the American woman has become the proverbial canary in the coal mine. It's letting us know that something has gone very wrong.

As a clinical nutritionist, over the past three decades I've worked with thousands of clients, mostly women, to effectively manage both their weight and their digestive issues. But it wasn't until 2011, when I cowrote *The Inside Tract: Your Good Gut Guide to Digestive Health* with Johns Hopkins gastroenterologist Gerard Mullin, that the connection between digestion and healthy weight became crystal clear to me. That book brought a parade of women with digestive issues to my private nutrition practice, most of whom had been trying unsuccessfully for years to drop those stubborn pounds. Sometimes it was the unruly gut that was their biggest complaint, typically, a not-so-merry-go-round of constipation, diarrhea, gas, and bloating given the all-purpose label of irritable bowel syndrome. (You can take an IBS self-diagnosis test offered by the American College of Gastroenterology at http://gi.org/acg-institute/ibs-test/.) Sometimes it was just the weight. What was staring me in the face was that Irritable Bowel and what I now call Irritable Weight were usually two faces of the same underlying problem. With some of these clients, I'm working to overcome a serious chronic condition. But for most of them, and for probably the majority of people reading this book, the digestive symptoms come and go. They're a hassle, to be sure, but they're also telling us, screaming at us sometimes, that the body is not being properly nourished by the right foods in the right ways. Your digestion and your weight are coconspirators, chipping away at your wellness.

SWIFT DIET DICTIONARY

Microbiome: The total collection of genes belonging to the bacteria that live inside our bodies and on our skin. These single-cell bacteria are at least ten times as numerous as human cells and most of them reside in the human gut.

Microbiota: The name given to the population of bacteria that live in the human gut, mostly in the colon or large intestine. In the past twenty or so years, we've discovered that the microbiota plays a major role in digestion, gut health and overall health, including weight control.

Gut Flora or **Microflora:** Same meaning as "microbiota" above. In the outside world, "flora" refers to plant life. Inside our gut, it refers to our resident gut bacteria.

Dysbiosis: A change in the composition of the gut bacteria that harms digestion or overall health. It might be brought on by a bad diet, a stressful lifestyle, an infection or a food allergy or sensitivity. Common gut symptoms of dysbiosis include bloating, excess gas, constipation and diarrhea.

The Swift Diet is the fruit of my work at three landmark centers of health and wellness in the Berkshires foothills of western Massachusetts. First, as the former director of nutrition at the famous Canyon Ranch health resort, then at my friend and colleague Dr. Mark Hyman's Ultra-Wellness Center and more recently at the Kripalu Center for Yoga and Health, I've refined an approach that emphasizes delicious whole foods.

It's "flexitarian," mostly veggies with both plant and lean animal protein and a limited amount of whole grains, fruit and anti-inflammatory fats and oils. Over and over again, I've seen a laundry list of debilitating symptoms cleared up—bloated bellies, constipated bellies, joint pain, troublesome skin—and my clients lose the weight. Weight gain and weight loss are influenced by a number of factors—all of which I'll discuss in this book—but what I've learned, and what I incorporate into the Swift Diet, is that when we eat to heal the gut, and we make some basic gut-friendly lifestyle and stress-reduction adjustments, we address virtually all of them. The road to healing runs through the gut. Heal the gut, lose the weight—that's been my experience and my credo for a long time. Only now, thanks to the research biologists, we have the scientific insights that allow us to better understand what's going on at the microscopic level.

The Microbiome Revolution

The scientific world has undergone a revolution in the way it understands the gastrointestinal tract, specifically the role played by the bacteria that live there. They're called either the "microbiome," referring to their total package of genes, or the "microbiota" (in plain English, "small life"), referring to the organisms themselves. We've known for about twenty years that the bacteria living in our colon break down the fiber that we get from plant sources—vegetables, fruits, legumes, nuts, seeds—which would otherwise be indigestible. What we've only just recently appreciated is that if the microbiota are not being properly attended to—if they're not being fed enough plant fiber or if they're being indiscriminately wiped out by the overuse of antibiotics or if they're damaged over time by excessive amounts of stress hormones—a Pandora's box of bad things gets opened up. Weight, digestion and the workings of the immune system can go haywire.

One of the nation's most eminent microbiologists, Dr. Martin Blaser, believes that the nation's damaged microbiota is likely a major factor driving the rise of obesity and autoimmune disorders over the past several decades, and his lab at New York University is hard at work amassing the experimental evidence to prove the hypothesis. Just this year, he's laid out his case to a general audience in his *Missing Microbes: How the Overuse of Antibiotics Is Fueling Our Modern Plagues.*

In the past few years, the research has moved from cells under the microscope and mouse studies to real-live humans struggling with their weight. In a landmark 2013 study published in the prestigious journal *Nature*, a French team tracked two groups of subjects, 169 obese people and 123 leans ones.

The lean group, it turned out, had more bacteria at work in their guts and more different strains than their heavier counterparts. They were less likely to gain weight over the nine years of the study and less likely to develop the most common chronic diseases, such as heart disease and type 2 diabetes. Well, you might say, the lean group was just born lucky. But in a second study published in the same issue of *Nature* by some of the same researchers, 49 subjects who were overweight were put on a lower-calorie, higher-fiber diet for six weeks. "We really wanted to have this fiber enrichment so the study subjects ate a good amount of vegetables and fruits," says Professor Karine Clément, one of the study coauthors and the director of ICAN, the Institute of Cardiometabolism and Nutrition in Paris.

Not only did the participants lose weight, but the community of bacteria in their guts became richer and more diverse; in other words, it more closely resembled the bacteria in the people who were naturally lean. Their metabolism and digestion had shifted to support their weight-loss efforts.

Think about that. We all know that some people seem more prone to gaining weight than others. (Believe me, I know. I struggled with my weight for years, and even now I still have to be conscious of how and what I eat to maintain my comfort weight zone.) And we've learned that our genetic inheritance plays a role here—over fifty genes have been identified that are associated with obesity. All of which sounds depressing—we can't change our genes, so if we've been dealt a bad genetic hand, we're simply out of luck. What the revolution in microbiology is telling us is that we *can* change the genes in our microbiome, and that will have an enormous effect on how we look and feel. Because the life cycle of single-celled bacteria is fantastically speeded up compared to the human one, making some straightforward adjustments to your diet and lifestyle will cause the helpful bacteria to increase in number and diversity, and the harmful ones to recede, in a very short period of time. (The biologists call this "exerting selective evolutionary pressure.")

While upgrading diet and lifestyle choices will always be the surest, most sustainable way to lose weight, there looks to be another way of leveraging the power of the microbiome, this one involving probiotics. Probiotics are friendly bacteria from the outside world that we consume, either in the form of fermented foods (we'll get to that in Chapter 4) or supplements (in Chapter 5). In a study published in December 2013 in the *British Journal of Nutrition*, Canadian researchers first put 150 overweight men and women on a diet and then on a weight-maintenance program. Half the study subjects also took two daily probiotic capsules of a bacterial strain similar to one found in yogurt; half did not. The women (but not the men) taking the probiotics lost considerably more weight than their counterparts who didn't, 9.7 pounds compared to 5.7 pounds. The women on the probiotics continued to lose weight during the maintenance phase, for a total weight loss that was twice as much as that of the other women. These are early days in trying to figure how to engineer probiotics to reliably get these kinds of effects, but the potential, for women anyway, is breathtaking!

The 4-week Swift Plan

The Canadian researchers got those results with a 12-week diet and 12-week maintenance phase. The French researchers measured important changes in the gut bacteria after a 6-week diet. In my clinical experience, I've found that four weeks is plenty of time to reap the initial benefits of eating and living in tune with your gut. And so, in the coming chapters, I'll take you through the principles of a microbiotically aligned diet and lifestyle, then guide you through the 4-week Swift Plan, the template for a healthy *and* pleasurable lifetime journey.

And no matter how sophisticated the underlying biology, the diet guidelines couldn't be simpler: take out the fattening and toxic foods in your diet that wreak havoc on your microbiota and put in the delicious, nutritious foods that support it. The path has got to be simple when you intend to stay on it forever. That's why the current vogue for complicated multiphase diets has never made any sense to me. I'd say that about 90 percent of the women I see in my practice are refugees from these diets.

But they're undaunted. They're willing to commit one more time. By the time they, and the readers of *The Swift Diet*, have completed the 4-week Plan, they will have learned how to tune in to their own "nutritional wisdom." Was the food they ate today mostly whole foods (veggies, fruits, beans, nuts, fish and lean animal protein), with little or no processed foods? Did most of it come from plants, not animals? Were the fruits and vegetables "color-coded," that is, did they come in a range of colors? Did the dishes they prepare have tasty and health-protecting herbs and spices? Did they have a fermented food dish? (More on all of this in Chapter 4.)

What happens when you embrace this approach? Let me briefly run down the list. Weight loss—yes. How much and how fast will depend on your unique metabolism and where you begin the journey—your current weight and your eating and exercise (or lack thereof) habits. I've worked with clients who've lost fifteen pounds in four weeks and those who've lost five pounds. I honor both because each person is metabolically unique and I know they'll reach their goals at their own pace. How about the bloat? The excess fluid that your system is carrying, especially around the waist, shrinks or disappears. Those annoying and sometimes absolutely enervating symptoms of digestive upset subside. Energy and mood lift. Those seemingly uncontrollable food cravings, especially for the sweet stuff, become manageable or sometimes barely noticeable. Skin clears up. Muscle and joint aches and pains subside. I've seen it all, on a regular basis, and not only in my private nutrition clients who commit to the four weeks. Over the past seven years, I've developed and led workshops on digestive health, detoxification and "integrative" weight loss at Kripalu in Stockbridge, Massachusetts, the nation's largest residential yoga and health center. The clients there commit to an "immersion" experience but they're free to eat and exercise as much or as little as they want. And I've seen the kinds of results I've just described begin to take hold over the course of a single workshop—that's five days!

Don't get me wrong. I'm disturbed by inflated or frankly bogus health or weight-loss claims (or, as I like to call it, "cure-isma"). I'm a research maven. When I'm not working with clients, I'm likely to be surfing academic journals, tracking the latest research online. For more than a decade, I've organized an annual Food As Medicine conference, which brings together doctors, nutritionists and other health care professionals from all over the country to discuss and disseminate the latest nutritional breakthroughs. But as strongly as I'm committed to what's called "evidence-based medicine," I also recognize that there is such a thing as "practice-based evidence." Another way of putting it is "clinical wisdom."

The beauty of the Swift Diet is that the white-coat lab research perfectly dovetails with the results I get with my clients. It's a "diet," not in the sense of temporary calorie deprivation (the "white-knuckle" approach usually just leads to yo-yo weight loss and regain), but in the sense of aligning the way you eat and live with how your gut actually functions. And it's "Swift" because, well, that's my name and, more fundamentally, because the microbiota respond so swiftly to positive changes in diet and lifestyle, wasting no time delivering those benefits in weight, digestive health and overall well-being. Those bacteria do move incredibly quickly. In another 2014 *Nature* study, the composition of the gut microbiome changed dramatically within four days of the subjects switching from all-animal-products diet to a vegetarian one, and vice versa.

Do Calories Count?

Before I introduce you to my five-step MENDS program that is, forgive the expression, the guts of the Swift Diet and this book, let me clear up a fundamental confusion about diet and weight loss. Especially if you're a veteran of calorie-counting diets in the past, you may be asking, "Kathie, are you saying that as long as I'm eating the right kind of gut-friendly foods, I can eat as much as I want, that calories don't matter?" It's a big question. On one side, you have experts, especially coming from the alternative medicine world, who are now saying exactly that, that it's all about the quality of the calories and how they interact with the microbiome, indeed with all of the genes in our body, bacterial and human. The quantity of calories is no big deal. On the other side, a lot of mainstream doctors and nutritionists still hold to the traditional view that weight gain and loss are simply a numbers game, so-called calories in/calories out. Consume more calories than you burn, through physical activity and just being alive, and the excess gets stored as fat. The inevitable prescription: "Eat less, exercise more."

Guess what? It's both—both the quality and the quantity of the calories you eat count. But I'll go further than that. The number of calories and the nutritional value of those calories are, in a practical sense, two ways of looking at the same thing. The vegetables that constitute the bulk of the Swift Diet are low in calories, so you don't have to count calories when you follow my meal plans and recipes. Caloric restriction is built into the ingredients and portion sizes, as is the nourishment, for you and your microbiome! The single element that glues together these two conceptions of food is fiber. The Swift Diet is "holistic," integrating all of the important aspects of weight loss and digestive health, including lifestyle and stress-reducing mind-body exercises. I like to say, healthy weight loss is about learning to better digest your life. But if you had to pin me down on the single most important nutritional element, it would be dietary fiber.

When we consume plant-based foods, the fiber in these foods is high-volume—it helps trigger a feeling of fullness, or satiety, simply by taking up more room in our stomachs. The bacteria that break down the fiber in the gut produce a compound, acetate, that sends the brain a similar fullness message. As well, fiber slows down the process of digestion. That means, the body breaks down the carbohydrates into fuel that it can use, glucose, more slowly. When our blood sugar levels are more stable, our bodies don't have to produce as much of the hormone insulin to escort the glucose into our muscle and liver cells. The net result: we stay full longer and avoid those spikes in blood sugar and insulin that cause "boom-bust" hunger—we eat a high-carb meal and then a big shot of insulin rapidly clears the sugar so one minute we're full and the next we're hungry. Put another way, the quality of the calories helps us limit the quantity.

When a client tells me after a few days on the program, "I can't believe it, Kathie; I'm not hungry anymore!" I know a fundamental metabolic shift has taken place. The fiber is doing its job: directly, by promoting fullness, and indirectly, by replacing a lot of the quick-digesting carbs and simple sugars that overstimulate insulin production and promote weight gain. Over time, chronic overproduction of insulin leads to insulin resistance—the pancreas makes more and more insulin and the muscle and liver cells pay less and less attention to it—which leads to more weight gain and, ultimately, to type 2 diabetes. In some people, these sugar-rush carbs activate pleasure circuits in the brain that invite food addiction. (I'll talk more about that in Chapter 3.)

Under the Microscope

But there's another dimension to the fiber story, and that returns us to the scientific frontier of the microbiome. Let's go under the microscope. For starters, the single-cell bacteria in our bodies outnumber our human cells more than 10 to 1, leading some biologists to suggest that we're not really human at all, not exactly, but rather a superorganism, a collection of species that add up to a communal whole. (You could think of your body as a coral reef!) Nowhere are the bacteria more numerous or more important than in the gut, congregated mostly in the last station in the digestive tract, the colon or large intestine.

The dietary fiber we consume in vegetables, fruits, legumes, nuts and seeds can't be digested by our own human cells. In the colon, the bacteria break it down for their own energy needs via fermentation, similar to the way bacteria ferment milk into yogurt. It's a bargain for both parties—we give the bacteria a place to live and a free lunch, and they in return create the friendly fermentation by-products that actually feed the cells of our colon and keep it healthy. They also produce important vitamins like B_{12}, biotin and vitamin K.

What happens if we don't feed the colon with a fiber-rich whole-foods diet? The good bacteria that feed on fiber—the bifidobacteria and the lactobacilli, to name two—decline in number and get pushed aside by potentially nasty, opportunistic bugs, unfriendly bacteria and often yeast and parasites, which can team up to cause those distressing digestive symptoms. And with fewer good bacteria handling fermentation duties, fewer by-products are being created to feed the cells that line the wall of the colon. The wall that separates the gut from the rest of the body grows porous over time, allowing bits and pieces of harmful microorganisms to leak into the bloodstream. We call this "increased intestinal permeability" or "leaky gut syndrome" and it can trigger low-grade inflammation throughout the system, leading to insulin resistance, which means that extra calories get more readily stored as fat, driving weight gain.

What are the consequences of adding these pounds, mostly "visceral fat" that smothers our internal organs and pushes out the belly? The now larger, and possibly more numerous, fat cells send out inflammatory hormones into the bloodstream that drive more weight gain. (Biologists now regard our adipose tissue as the largest endocrine, that is, hormone-producing, gland in the body.) And the extra weight further unsettles the gut. Overweight people seem more likely to carry the bacterial species that are linked with leaky gut. (It wasn't a surprise when the French researchers found that lean and overweight people had very different-looking microbiomes.) So this is a vicious circle if there ever was one! I call it Irritable Weight. One of the world's leading microbiome scientists, Patrice Cani, at the Université Catholique de Louvain in Belgium, calls it "MicroObesity."

Researchers like Cani filled in a crucial part of the weight gain/weight loss puzzle. In the past, everyone locked into the idea that it was all about burning more calories. We had to keep the "fire" of metabolism burning brightly! Well, "calories out" *is* an important consideration—exercise, for instance, which I'll discuss in Chapter 6. But in my opinion, getting too caught up with "revving up the metabolism" has led to gimmicks like "belly-blasting" potions and creams, most of which are of dubious value, and "metabolic-boosting" supplements, some of which can be downright unsafe. Now, thanks to the microbiome scientists, we can appreciate that just as important as raising the fire of metabolism is *lowering* the fire of inflammation that affects the hormones, insulin first among them, that control how many of the calories we take in get burned for energy and how many get stored as fat.

Your Immune System: Good Gut Gone Wrong?

There's another important way that food impacts the gut bacteria, upsets digestion and can lead to weight gain. That's via the immune system and that's a story unto itself.

About 70 percent of the activity of the immune system takes place in the gut. The microbiome plays a crucial role, "tuning" the human immune system to distinguish friend from foe. Why would nature outsource such a big job, helping the body defend itself against external threat, to roughly one hundred trillion resident bacteria who aren't even remotely human? As with real estate (and we're dealing with digestive real estate here), the answer is, "Location, location, location." The digestive tract is the body's primary entry point for the outside world, in the form of food, with its collection of foreign proteins and germs, good, bad and indifferent. So that's where our "bugs" are: the gut contains somewhere between five hundred and one thousand different strains of bacteria that make up our microbiota. You can think of the entire digestive tract, from the mouth to the stomach to the small intestine to the large intestine or colon to the anus, as a single thirty-feet tube designed to bring the outside world into us, right through the very center of us. In this way, we can extract the nutrition we need under reasonably safe and controlled conditions, with all of the digesting, absorbing and, finally, excreting taking place in connecting chambers walled off from the rest of the body by a mucous lining. And our resident bacteria, because they are so numerous and they turn over so quickly—a population of gut bacteria can double their numbers in about twenty minutes—are uniquely well suited to form the immune system's rapid response team.

And sometimes things go wrong. Sometimes the human immune system, ill-served by a microbiome that's lacking in number and diversity, overreacts, which is what happens to people with a gluten sensitivity. The body treats one of the proteins in gluten like a foreign invader and mounts an inflammatory response. The upset is often felt in the gut, but because the gut and the brain are constantly sending chemical messages back and forth, symptoms like fatigue, "brain fog" and anxiety are common as well. The more unhappy and out-of-balance the gut bacteria—*dysbiosis* is the technical term—the more likely you'll suffer from these sometimes disabling food intolerances.

If you follow the major health stories in the media over the past few years, you know that, increasingly, inflammation is suspected as being a villain behind the most serious "diseases of aging": heart disease, type 2 diabetes, Alzheimer's and even cancer. It's paradoxical. Inflammation is the body's effort to respond to injury or infection by cordoning off the area and sending in specialized cells to clean up the damage. We couldn't survive without this biological response. However, while the body is quick to call out the troops, it's often not so good at calling them back. Considering how bound up the gut bacteria are in so many areas of our health, and the inflammatory processes that undermine them, some researchers are beginning to wonder whether, as the influential food writer Michael Pollan framed it in a *New York Times Magazine* cover story, "medical science may be on the trail of a Grand Unified Theory of Chronic Disease, at the very heart of which we will find the gut microbiome." The tools of microbiology and genomic sequencing seem to have brought us back to a place that the ancients might recognize. To the Indian sages who centuries ago codified Ayurveda, the Indian philosophy of medicine, *agni*, "the digestive fire," was the all-important measure of health. Hippocrates, the Greek father of Western medicine, famously said, "Let food be thy medicine, thy medicine shall be thy food."

Kathie's Story

These aren't just clinical or philosophical issues with me. I've lived it. When it comes to the microbiota and gut/weight health, you could say I was born with three strikes against me. I was a Caesarean preemie, bottle-fed and, as a sickly little kid, I spent a good chunk of my early years on antibiotics.

We don't come into the world with a developed microbiota, far from it. We live largely germ-free in the womb and then we acquire a bacterial starter kit as we pass through the birth canal when we're born, the basis for our gut's immune system. Then, as babies, if we're lucky, we consume breast milk. It's the perfect infant food to nourish the microbiota that will be needed when that baby grows into a toddler eating solid food.

None of this applied to me, a bottle-fed Caesarean, just as many of you will have missed out on the advantages of being breast-fed or being brought into this world via vaginal delivery, the best inoculation possible for a healthy start in life. Adding insult to injury were the medications I was prescribed for my problematic digestion, the antacids and the proton pump inhibitors (PPIs) that actually interfered with normal gut function. Worse still, the multiple courses of antibiotics I was given in my early years further depleted my gut bacteria, which probably contributed to the health issues I always seemed to be struggling with as a child: chronic ear infections, headaches and a very irritable bowel.

Work by microbiome pioneers like Dr. Blaser and anthropologist Jeff Leach, the cofounder of the American Gut Project, has established that the overuse of antibiotics—by some expert estimates, half of the antibiotics we consume are unnecessary or useless—is one of the prime causes of the depletion of the helpful bacteria in the American gut. Leach likens it to bombing your backyard with toxic chemicals: "You spray everything and it's the invading, opportunistic species that come back first." Dr. Blaser is currently doing research studying how a human microbiome, deprived of certain bacteria by antibiotics or simple lack of exposure to the bugs in the natural world, can throw off the communication between the gut and the hormones that regulate hunger. Some of us may be overeating because our brain isn't getting the message that we're full!

In any event, I survived my childhood. I was always outdoors, fairly athletic and I enjoyed OK health until I hit my early thirties when, as a busy wife and mother of two young children, I battled chronic fatigue syndrome. My husband, Dan, was at the time a U.S. Air Force pilot and when he was transferred to an air base in southern England, we were excited to be having a family adventure. The day before we left for the UK, I got hit by some sort of stomach bug and after that passed, I was laid low by an exhaustion that just wouldn't lift. I'd want so desperately to go on a bike ride with the kids that I would make myself do it and then wind up back in bed, totally wiped out. And since I couldn't exercise, my weight began to steadily creep up.

The military doctors diagnosed me with an autoimmune disease and wanted to send me back to the States for more advanced tests, but I was determined to figure things out for myself. It turned out the major culprit was all of the wheat-based foods I was eating, specifically the gluten protein that's in many grains and most definitely in the muesli I ate every morning with the kids, the whole-wheat sandwich I ate for lunch, the pasta I cooked for the family at dinner. It certainly was in those delicious scones that seemed to be everywhere I turned. I was feeding a sensitivity to gluten that in all likelihood was triggered by that stomach bug. Today, researchers understand that a bout of bacterial food poisoning or a stomach virus will often trigger a latent food sensitivity. But this was the eighties and almost no one had ever heard of gluten sensitivities. Eventually, with the help of intellectual mentors like Dr. Jeffrey Bland, the biochemist father of the "functional medicine" movement in the United States, I slowly figured things out. In a strange way, those early struggles were a gift. I have spent a career searching for—and then finding and developing—solutions for people burdened with weight and digestive problems.

In 1991, when my family and I moved to the Berkshires, the northwestern corner of Massachusetts, I became the director of nutrition at Canyon Ranch, the famous Tucson resort that had opened a new, luxurious spa in the town of Lenox. At the Ranch, I learned and then taught the importance of a whole life—including natural weight loss as a result of healthy, delicious meals as well as eating, moving and sleeping on a regular schedule.

I believed in the power of the right foods to heal and to manage weight. This was reflected in my own life, as I steadily cut back on the amount of animal protein my family and I ate and increased the amount of vegetables and completely switched over to gluten-free grains. Meals now are moderate portions, high in fiber and loaded with vitamins and minerals. And,

unlike many diets that separate the dieter from her family, this way of eating made the whole family healthier and brought us together for delicious
meals we all enjoyed. I was able to eat my way back to health and a healthy
weight, helped by daily exercise once I had my normal energy back.

When I saw the results in my life and in my clients' lives, I became
unstoppable. I helped persuade the food development team at the Ranch to
jettison their signature "60/20/20" formula (that is, carbs, fats, proteins)
to embrace something we called "nutritional intelligence." While everyone's metabolism is unique, every woman can exercise her nutritional
intelligence to lose weight by becoming mindful of portion size and building diets around lower-calorie, fiber-and-nutrient-dense food, especially
veggies.

I formed a kind of "brain trust" with the medical directors at Canyon
Ranch, health pioneers and authors Dr. Mark Liponis and Dr. Mark
Hyman. Our medical/nutritional team spearheaded an "ultra-preventative"
approach to health and vitality that was ahead of its time. Years later, when
Dr. Hyman started up his own clinic in Lenox, the UltraWellness Center, I
followed as the head of the nutrition department. We embraced a "food is
medicine" philosophy, fine-tuning meal plans to help heal a range of health
problems, like type 2 diabetes and IBS, with which conventional medicine
had had little success.

While I continue to work with Mark at the UltraWellness Center, for
the past six years I've devoted most of my time, outside my own private
nutritional practice, to the workshops I lead at the Kripalu Center and
around the country. It's a two-way street. I teach my students about the
microbiome and how they can leverage it to reach their healthy-living
goals. And, in turn, I'm routinely blown away by the transformations I've
seen in them that can take place in a few short days, how mind-body practices like yoga and qigong can calm their stress levels and strengthen their
resolve. I strongly believe, and a raft of studies backs me up, that these
movement therapies are a kind of invitation to my students to enter into a
different relationship with their bodies. A body in need of balance needn't
be the enemy but more like a dear old friend—accepted and capable of

surprising you in positive ways. Compassion and nonjudgment are such beautiful antidotes to the self-blame that so often undercuts the commitment to healthy weight.

In addition to my workshops, I do nutritional consulting for a local financial company in the Berkshires. Currently, the small group of women I'm working with there have formed their own weight and lifestyle-reboot group. These are overweight middle-aged women who work hard at their office jobs to help support their families. They've embraced the whole foods, mostly plant-based diet, and I've got them doing a modicum of exercise and a few basic qigong practices, which they love. As of this writing, they have been on the program for eight months and between them they've lost more than one hundred pounds. They feel fantastic. And so do I. I eat and exercise and make use of stress-reducing techniques the same way my clients do, the same way I trust my readers will. And at sixty, this is the best I've ever felt in my entire life. I feel blessed to have grown into this knowledge about the healing power of food and for the chance to share it with others.

The MENDS Approach

I've integrated my clinical and my personal experiences with the latest microbiome research to create MENDS, the five-step program that is the backbone of the Swift Diet. There is nothing here that is intrinsically difficult or complex. But we all recognize that changing old habits can feel daunting—"Where do I begin? What do I have to change first?" With that in mind, I'm devoting one chapter, Chapter 7, to a 4-week Swift Plan that takes readers by the hand into this new world of delicious whole foods, day by day, meal by meal. The message here couldn't be more empowering. With some straightforward modifications to the way we eat, and some smart lifestyle tweaks, we can change the composition of the microbial community inside us. Beginning that first month, MENDS and the Swift Diet will pay out weight and health dividends over the course of your entire life.

M—Mind Your Digestion

Digestion actually begins in the mind. That is why I start my program here. The hungry brain sends out messages to orchestrate the production of enzymes and acids that the body will use to process the food. Our GI (gastrointestinal) tract is packed with neurotransmitters like serotonin and dopamine—"the second brain." Too much stress can upset the balance of bacteria in our gut, which contributes to the IBS-type problems that many of us are familiar with when we feel like we're under the gun. And when cortisol, our primary stress hormone, goes into overdrive, that actually promotes fat gain around the middle, the last thing we want. Daily, it seems, researchers are making breakthroughs to unravel the brain-belly connection.

If a stressed-out brain can make life miserable for the belly by upsetting digestion and adding on pounds, the mind can heal the damage and take off the weight. In this first M section of my program, I introduce you to the basics of eating mindfully, including: giving the "cephalic" (from the Greek, "in the head") digestion system the time it needs to properly digest food without irritation or inflammation; engaging with your body's inner sense of satiety or fullness; and spacing meals so that the gut has time to cleanse itself and prepare for the next intake of food (no more "grazing" throughout the day!).

In this M step, I also cover "mind" in a broader way, addressing the fears and anxieties that can trigger the stress response, interfering with healthy digestion and encouraging weight gain. The first fear to defuse is the fear of food itself: don't make food the enemy. The flip side is the fear that eating healthy means giving up the most satisfying food pleasures—so not true! The fear of hunger is the elephant in the room. I explain how mindful eating partnered with a digestion-friendly diet translates to weight loss without hunger.

In this chapter, I'll also introduce some simple "mindfulness" practices that do double duty: not only do they lower stress hormones levels, which, unchecked, can derange the microbiome and upset digestion; they encourage a focus on what's really important, to help ensure that you stay the healthy weight and digestion course.

E—Eliminate the "Problem" Foods

I've created a MicroMenaces list of foods that disrupt the microbiome and drive weight and gut problems. I unapologetically take a hard line here, aggressively cutting back on processed, refined carbohydrates, such as breakfast cereals, crackers and pastas, and in their place substituting limited amounts of gluten-free whole grains, such as quinoa and buckwheat. These refined carb foods deliver a double whammy. They can trigger systemic inflammation, which then promotes weight gain. And the high number of calories is more than the body can burn, so that excess gets shuttled into fat storage. Researchers speculate that our overconsumption of these refined carbs is the number one reason why our society suffers from obesity and diseases of aging like heart disease, dementia and type 2 diabetes.

Next on the list are the unhealthy fats: trans fats and too much saturated and omega-6 fats. There is a growing body of research showing that excess dietary fat, in particular saturated fat, can promote weight and digestive problems via leaky-gut syndrome, which I'll explain in some detail. Mass-produced vegetable oils like corn oil and soy oil, genetically modified and often processed to contain harmful trans fats, are another big concern.

Now we come to "problematic protein." Red meat in particular is rich in protein that can create troublesome by-products when it's broken down by the bacteria in the gut. And industrially processed meat of any kind usually contains supplemental hormones, antibiotics, and even stress compounds produced by animals raised in cruel, crowded conditions. Yes, there is room for lean, clean meat and poultry, but only in limited amounts. Study after study has confirmed that a mostly plant-based diet is the healthiest way to eat.

The last major group, and it occupies a number of slots on my Micro-Menace list, is food containing specific "irritants." In some people, hard-to-digest food components, such as the gluten in grains and the lactose in dairy, can upset the digestive system and cause a host of nagging symptoms. I'll also discuss how to handle specific vegetables, fruits and legumes that are packed with healthy fibers, and how to rebuild digestive resilience by gradually introducing these foods to bring the microbiota back into balance.

N—Nourish the Body, and the Belly

As the microbiome scientists have confirmed, eating for gut health and weight loss isn't just about avoiding certain foods that can cause problems; it's about embracing a much broader spectrum of foods that can help resolve them. Foods like arugula, broccoli, winter squash, and lentils are the stars of my MicroMenders list. These non-starchy vegetables, starchy vegetables and legumes are "prebiotic"—that is, the fiber in them feeds the strains of gut bacteria that we know are especially important for the health of the colon and our overall health. They're one-stop shopping: high in fiber, low in calories and rich in vitamins, minerals, and compounds called phytonutrients, which combat disease by tamping down inflammation and pumping up antioxidants. Wherever possible, I choose "wild foods" such as arugula and purple potatoes, which are close or identical to their plant ancestors and haven't had the nutrition bred out of them in the name of appearance or sweetness. Recently, there's been an explosion of interest in fermented foods, such as sauerkraut, kimchi, yogurt and kefir, which deliver their own dose of bacteria that helps our native gut bacteria strains do their job. In this chapter, you'll learn more about fermented foods (what you think may be fermented often isn't) and how to integrate these cultured goodies into your daily diet.

D—Dietary Supplements

While nothing can or should take the place of reforming diet to tackle weight loss and digestive health, supplements have their place. Probiotics, supplements that contain billions of units of live-culture bacteria, are powerful tools in my toolbox. By supporting the "resident" microbiota, these "transient" bugs can help calm digestive ills, and there is research to indicate that they may offer a meaningful weight-loss boost as well. The recent Canadian study that found that a daily probiotic supplement doubled weight loss for a group of women over a six-month period has opened some eyes. I'll discuss how to be a smart probiotic shopper and how to decipher the different brands, bacterial strains and dosages.

Fiber supplements offer a healthy three-for-the-price-of-one: they promote regularity, they are the best natural appetite suppressant we have and they have some ability to feed the microbiota. In Chapter 5, I'll discuss various fiber supplement options, including psyllium and konjac root.

I'll also discuss broad-spectrum digestive enzymes that can be useful for people who, because of age or illness, are having problems extracting nutrition from the food they eat. I'll also cover supplemental superstars like vitamin D, omega-3 fatty acids and magnesium, as well as some nutritional and herbal remedies for common digestive ills.

S—Sustaining Practices

This final MENDS chapter (Chapter 6) will be devoted to simple, eminently doable lifestyle tweaks, bringing the way you live your everyday life into alignment with your intention to heal the belly and lose the weight. Exercise and sleep are two crucial areas.

I'll introduce readers to an expanding new research field that connects poor-quality or insufficient sleep with obesity and digestive dysfunction. These studies have found that going to bed late or not getting enough sleep raises cortisol, insulin, and blood sugar levels, which upset the gut bacteria and keep the appetite pump primed. My simple SOS (Swift Optimal Sleep) plan will help ensure seven to nine hours of sleep a night.

Exercise defuses excess stress and stress-related digestive problems, and the calorie burn and metabolic boost it provides are crucial for maintaining healthy weight loss. I'll present a structured exercise guide to get the occasional exerciser or non-exerciser moving. The emphasis here is on the practical. It's got to be convenient and fun enough so that you stay with it. I'll also pay special attention to spending time in nature, whether it's snatching a moment of meditative silence or vigorous hiking, and how that can recharge our emotional and weight-loss batteries. Finally, I'll go deeper into some of the stress-reducing techniques I touch on in Chapter 2. In Chapter 6, I'll provide the reader with an entrée to both yoga and a related mind-body tradition from ancient China, qigong. When I studied the research literature on weight loss and yoga and qigong, the positive results weren't a revelation but a confirmation of what I and many of my clients experience every day.

Whether it's sleep, exercise, or stress-reducing mind-body techniques, the organizing principle of the chapter is: finding a pleasing and satisfying rhythm to your day. As I'll explain, we want to live in tune with the body's circadian rhythms, what some researchers are now calling our "chronobiology."

The power of the MENDS program is the whole package. Truly, it's about "digesting your life."

"As Above, So Below"

What I love about MENDS and the microbiome-attuned approach to weight loss and digestive health is not only that it works but *how* it works. Most weight-loss plans begin and end with a sense of me: "I want to look this way, feel that way." That motivation is important, and the Swift Diet will tap into it, wisely. But if you really embrace it, the Swift Diet enlarges your sense of "me." Your well-being depends on keeping a community of microorganisms working with you, not against you. And just like any other community we care to think of, it can become dysfunctional or, in gut language, dysbiotic. It has to be brought back into balance.

There's a saying that sometimes pops up in esoteric literature: "As above, so below." In other words, the microcosm is a reflection of the macrocosm. I can't think of anywhere where that is more obviously and literally true than in the humble gut. The inflamed American gut, responsible for weight gain and digestive unhappiness, is a reflection of a sugar-driven junk-food culture that values convenience and corporate profits above all else. On a global scale, our hunger for beef consumes an unconscionable amount of the world's natural resources, contributing to climate change and a loss of ecosystems that are rich in species both visible and invisible to the human eye. The big lesson of ecology is that less diversity means less resilience in the face of external threat, and that's true whether we're talking about a forest, a coral reef or your gut.

This shrinking biodiversity has implications that go beyond weight and digestive health. Maybe you've heard of the "hygiene hypothesis"? This is the idea that as we're exposed to fewer microbes in the soil and water in the natural world—and as we prune back our own gut microbes with processed-food diets and the overzealous use of antibiotics—our immune system becomes less and less able to accurately assess external threats. We have fewer friendly bacteria on board to protect us from the relatively few who are not. It's our best working explanation as to why the rates of auto-immune diseases like asthma and Hashimoto's thyroiditis (low thyroid) have skyrocketed over the past several decades. We're "cleaner" but we're sicker. To take one example, Swedish researchers tracked a group of forty-seven children from infancy to age seven. The fewer types of bacteria they had in their guts, the more likely they were to develop autoimmune diseases or allergies such as asthma, hay fever and eczema. In 2013, the World Allergy Organization published a position paper that made a forceful case that less diversity in the macro world leads to less diversity in the micro world in our gut. As above, so below!

OK, we're not going to restore natural habitats or solve climate change tomorrow. But by choosing to eat a mostly plant-based diet, we are voting with our forks, pushing the macroscopic world in the right direction one micron at a time. We can live and eat in a mindful way, in tune with the microcosm of our own gut bacteria. And if there's only so much we can do to protect ourselves from environmental pollution—for instance, the toxic chemicals in our plastics and household products—there's everything we can do to stop the internal toxins that build up in our bodies when we eat foods that inflame the gut.

Not long ago, I was taking part in a meeting where the doctors were presenting these depressing stories about susceptible clients getting sick because of environmental factors beyond their control. An atmosphere of doom and gloom was settling over the room and finally I couldn't take it anymore. "Wait a minute," I said. "The average American only gets ten to fifteen grams of nourishing prebiotic fiber a day. If we can increase that, we can make people a lot more resilient to whatever toxins we are exposed to!"

Another recent meeting comes to mind. I was giving a presentation to a group of health care professionals on the importance of the gut on everything from weight loss to energy to skin health. Afterward, an MD came up to me in tears. She was distraught that there was so much information out there that she could have used to help her patients had she only been aware of it. I told her not to be so hard on herself. Now was her time to learn and integrate these concepts into her dermatology practice. That reaffirmed to me that I was on the right path. Even very caring, intellectually curious doctors were in the dark. And I was in a position to synthesize the research on the microbiome, which has exploded over the past few years, with what I knew worked from my thirty years in clinical nutrition. I could translate that science into a practical guide for women who were committed to achieve healthy weight and heal the gut.

ROOT CAUSES OF DIGESTIVE DISTRESS

Bottle feeding instead of breast feeding

Caesarean section birth

Chronic, unremitting stress

Circadian rhythm disruption

Food-borne illnesses

Infections

Loss of microbiome biodiversity

Overuse of medications (especially antacids, antibiotics, nonsteroidal anti-inflammatory meds, etc.)

Poor diet

Sedentary lifestyle

Sleep deprivation

Ultraclean hygiene

Chapter 2

M: MIND YOUR DIGESTION

Anna

Anna, a fifty-year-old attorney from Boston, is a disciplined, analytical person. When she came to me, she'd done a lot of research on various diets in an effort to get a handle on the twenty pounds she couldn't seem to shake, as well as the overall fatigue she felt was holding her back in her work and her life. (Some intermittent IBS symptoms didn't help either.) Anna and I were discussing how to modify her eating plan when she got very anxious. I don't think she even realized it, but every time I brought up a particular food, she would say, "I read that I should keep away from that kind of food for such-and-such reason." She was my "keep-away" client. After about the fifth "keep-away," I paused and said, "Anna, can I ask you, is there someone or something that you're trying to keep away in your life?" Well, that turned into a very emotional session. So often it happens that emotional issues and anxiety get bound up in the effort to lose weight. We talked about her life as a whole—what made her happy, what didn't. I encouraged Anna to work with a therapist who could support her and explore mind-body techniques to soothe her nervous system. I prescribed a sabbatical from surfing the Web for nutrition articles. Instead of her spending a precious hour of her day reading

about the latest food or nutrient that might do her harm, we strate-
gized about finding joy! Anna loved to dance but hadn't in years, so
she joined a Zumba dance class at her local gym and made some new
friends. We worked on integrating meditation into her day, which
helped her tremendously. As she began to unwind by degrees over the
following months, she was able to integrate the diet changes that we
were able to discuss in a more open, less fearful way. She finally lost
the twenty pounds she'd wanted to shed for years.

SELF-INQUIRY BOX

1. Do you think, in your heart of hearts, that losing weight and keeping it off will be too hard, even impossible?
2. Have you ever caught yourself thinking about food as the enemy, the thing that frustrates your weight and health goals?
3. Have you noticed a connection between your mood, your gut and your weight? That low mood and digestive and weight issues sometimes clump together?

I t might strike you as odd that I'm beginning the first step of the MENDS program with a story that really isn't about food. In fact, it's about *not* thinking about food!

There is some amazing new science about how the microbiome directly influences the brain, including how the brain regulates appetite and digestion. In one study, eating yogurt, which is filled with probiotic bacteria, even changed the way the brain lights up on a brain-imaging study. But I want to begin this "Mind" chapter by addressing the ideas, and the emotions bound up in those ideas, that people commonly have about rebooting their diet and lifestyle to achieve and maintain healthy weight. Take Anna, for example. She couldn't begin to deal with her weight and gut issues until she turned down the volume on the anxiety buzzing through her, much of it triggered by her relationship with food.

Of course, I've had clients who wanted to dive into the meal plans right away, what they couldn't and could eat. And I can't *stop* you from skipping to the next two chapters, "Eliminate" and "Nourish," which are exactly about that. But I can tell you what often happened to my in-a-hurry clients. Everything goes great, for a while, and then the new-project shine wears off and old familiar emotional patterns reassert themselves. Emotions have real physiological consequences, namely, stress hormones orchestrated in the brain that have big effects in the gut and on weight loss. Like the song says, "Free your mind, and the rest will follow," especially the gut!

The fears and anxieties that can accompany committing to a healthy weight-loss program are insidious because, more often than not, they lie half-buried in our psyche. They sap our confidence, our ability to see ourselves as strong people able to make lasting changes in our lives, and yet often we're barely aware they're there. But if we can bring these fears into the light of the day and examine them rationally, usually they'll shrink in importance. You've probably heard some version of this "name it, own it" positive psychology before. It really does work.

Fear of Food

Anna is hardly the only client I've had who sabotaged herself by worrying *too* much about what she eats. The phenomenon has even been measured in research settings. In 2013, a group of New Zealand social scientists studied a group of three hundred people who were asked if eating a piece of chocolate cake would make them feel guilty or happy. Followed up eighteen months later, the minority who were guilty eaters had gained more weight than the majority who could allow themselves to enjoy a treat. Guilt, besides not being a lot of fun, is a setup for weight gain! In a similar vein, American researchers culled through questionnaires given to over five thousand people and identified seven distinct eating styles that were associated with overeating. One of the seven styles that women were far more prone to than men: Food Fretting.

I know, it sounds paradoxical. If you're trying to lose weight, why wouldn't the fear of food be a good thing? But it's not. Instead of building up your resolve, ultimately you'll undermine it. The anxiety about what you can and can't eat and what the wrong foods might do to you creates a constant tension that can suck the joy out of life. It also increases levels of the stress hormone cortisol, which can increase the hunger for a sugar quick fix, which in turn increases insulin levels, which promotes fat storage. Your strongest ally in a lifelong sustained weight-loss program is the self-trust and self-confidence that comes from embracing life, not trying to keep it at arm's length. Being able to take pleasure in food, and to share that pleasure with loved ones, should be a big part of that.

In Anna's case, a Zumba class helped her to begin to be able to break down the fearfulness that was keeping her in her shell, trapped in a failed weight-loss program that amounted to an ever-expanding list of "thou shall nots." I have another client, Rebecca, who suffers from gastroesophageal reflux disease, or GERD. She had become so fearful of food that she'd whittled her diet down to about six things she'd permit herself to eat. But she mentioned to me that once every few months, in the course of an afternoon of shopping, she would have lunch with her girlfriends and then, and only then, she wouldn't suffer from gastric reflux, no matter what she ate. I wrote her a "prescription" on the spot: once a week, have lunch with at least one girlfriend and let go of what's "good" or "bad" for you.

Fear of Giving Up Pleasure

A lot of my clients aren't as good at self-denial as Anna is. In fact, they're in love with the tempting pleasures of sugary, fatty processed foods. Life is tough enough. How, they wonder, are they going to get through it without the sweet release? This fear has a real basis. Social scientists, and any good student of human nature, know that willpower is limited and most people simply aren't capable of denying themselves indefinitely what they truly yearn for, one major reason why ultra-low-calorie diets, whatever their short-term success, rarely pay off in sustained weight loss. The Swift Diet is about shifting what you want, not denying it. When you become familiar with the Swift Plan recipes and meal plans, built on fresh vegetables and fruits and not requiring much more prep time than the old processed foods, your taste buds won't want to settle for a Luna Bar for lunch or a frozen entrée for dinner. Think back to when you were a child and the smile that crossed your face when you bit into a fresh peach in summertime. Commit to your sensory pleasure!

My friend Marc David, the founder of the Institute for the Psychology of Eating, tells a story about a client who lived on fast food. When Marc persuaded the client to slow down and concentrate on each Big Mac mouthful, he discovered that he actually disliked the taste and texture and changed his eating habits that day. (Yes, fast food is meant to be eaten fast.) Certainly the best-case scenario! Over the years, you may have conditioned your taste buds to respond to the lure of "hyper-palatable" processed foods. After a couple of weeks of not bombarding your taste buds with industrial concentrations of sugar, salt and fat, you'll be able to taste real food. Will you always prefer the taste of a serving of grapes to that of a Mrs. Field's chocolate-chip cookie? I can't promise that. But if you do fall off the wagon, temporarily—we all do—the cookie likely will taste too sweet.

Fear of Hunger

Hunger is often the elephant in the room here, one big reason why many diets come to grief. In Chapter 3, I'll go into detail about how you can counter physical hunger with a high-fiber diet. But hunger also has a strong emotional component. The fear of hunger is hardwired into us as a species. For most of our existence, humankind routinely experienced life-threatening (and all too often life-ending) periods of nutritional deprivation—game was scarce or the crops failed.

Today, in the developed world, the danger runs in the opposite direction. We can't experience the slightest intimation of hunger without being overwhelmed by a tsunami of empty-calorie junk food or beverages. Heaven forbid we should be more than a five-minute drive or stroll from the neighborhood coffee shop (where caffeine is often combined with sugary syrups and fluffy mountains of whipped topping). As a consequence, many people who struggle with their weight have lost the ability to feel comfortable in that "sweet spot" between fullness and hunger. They become anxious that hunger could overtake them at any moment. I often encourage my clients to "ride the hunger wave" and explore what physical hunger feels like, how it has a different quality than emotional hunger or hunger born out of habit or maybe even fatigue. When you're feeling hungry but your body doesn't really need food, you might want to plug yourself in to an engaging activity or try one of the relaxation exercises I introduce later in this chapter.

THE HUNGER/FULLNESS SCALE

Here's a simple tool I use with clients to help them sort out when it's an appropriate time to have a healthy meal or snack, turning attention to internal cues. Using the scale below, rate your physical hunger. You're shooting to hit that 3 "sweet spot."

The Hunger Scale

1 not physically hungry

3 moderate physical hunger/good time to eat

5 ravenous (uh-oh, anything goes!)

The Fullness Scale

1 not physically satisfied

3 gently satisfied/mind and belly feel sated

5 discomfort/too full

Fear of Failure

Probably the most common fear that emerges in the first few sessions with a new client is the fear of failure. No matter how strong your motivation to get healthy and lose weight (and check in with that motivation often!), don't be surprised to hear a voice in the back of your head whispering, "You couldn't do it last time. What makes you think this time is going to be any different?"

You know what? Honor those past attempts! I encourage you to see them not as failures but as experiments that yielded valuable information about what worked and what didn't, which you can put to use moving forward. The psychologist James Prochaska at the University of Rhode Island has devoted his academic career to understanding how we make major behavioral changes. He found that people who succeeded at changing the big things, like quitting smoking or drinking, went through early stages of "contemplation" and "preparation" before they were ready to make the big change. And they rarely got it right the first time. They sometimes even failed multiple times before they learned the necessary lessons and created the necessary momentum to succeed.

Consider the statistics that tell us that the majority of American women have tried to lose weight in their lives. If you're reading this book, you probably have your own database of past experiences to draw on. So, change the narrative. Shift it from, "Why did I fail?" (i.e., "What's wrong with me?") to *"What did I learn?"* It's time to shed that guilt that cloaks your weight-loss history.

TAKE NOTE

Visit a stationery shop or bookstore and look for a nice notebook or journal to record your day-to-day experiences with the Swift Diet. Buy one whose look speaks to you and that's small enough to fit into a purse or backpack. Keep it by your bed and, if this works for you, carry it with you during the day. Use it to devote a few minutes each morning to setting your intention. Do this for a week and then, after that, for as long as it feels useful. You might write something like: "I will pause to taste each bite today." Or "I will find sweetness in living today." And write down your fears and resistances, from the general—"I am afraid I will binge again"—to the specific—"I have a lunch date and am worried about the menu temptations."

ART (AND FOOD) THERAPY

This exercise might sound a little contrived, but I've used it for years with my private clients and in my workshops and it never fails to generate surprising and revealing results. Collect a blank sheet of paper and some colored pens and give yourself five minutes of quiet time. First, close your eyes and think about the concept of food, what it means to you. Open your eyes and draw a picture of an image or a memory that came up. I've had people draw prison bars or a stressful scene from childhood, like parents fighting at the family dinner table. I've also received lovely pictures of vegetable gardens, a visual representation of how these clients would like to be eating. Let it sink in and write an entry in your journal about what you think your picture means. What do you see? What perceptions do you want to shed or embrace? This discovery process is an important part of consciously setting your intention and laying the foundation for lasting weight loss and a healthy relationship to food.

Digesting with Your Brain

Let's move from the level of conscious thought to the brain that gives rise to it. The brain and gut are so tightly wired together, scientists now sometimes refer to the gut as the body's "second brain." We all understand this intuitively. It's embedded in the language—"butterflies in the stomach," "gut feeling," "going with your gut." But when we understand something about the physiology of the "gut-brain axis" and how our behavior affects it, we can make simple changes that allow us to work with our digestion instead of fighting it, enhancing health and weight loss in the bargain.

Digestion actually begins in the head. We call the first phase of digestion "cephalic," from the Greek, meaning "from the head." It kicks in when we think about food or a tasty meal. The sheer anticipation stimulates the production of salivary enzymes in the mouth that begin to break down the carbohydrates in our food. The saliva itself is a lubricant that ensures a smooth trip down the short, muscular tube of the esophagus.

Here is the way the system works. The food moves down the esophagus into the stomach, a balloon-like muscular bag that breaks the food into much smaller particles, physically squeezing it and secreting enzymes and powerful gastric acids. The stomach then slowly pours the processed contents of the meal, now a liquid called chyme, which has the consistency of a smoothie, into the small intestine, where most of the work of digestion takes place. Assisted by the pancreas, which secretes digestive enzymes, and the gall bladder, which contributes bile, the small intestine breaks down the carbohydrates, proteins and fats in the chyme into their most basic components.

If the stomach resembles a factory, with its nonstop pulverizing and chemical baths, the small intestine is something closer to the undersea world of Jacques Cousteau, home to exotic-looking bulbous structures and beautiful in its own way. In the small intestine, some twenty-one feet of tubing is folded in on itself, but the surface area is much greater than even that suggests. Completely flattened out, it would cover a tennis court! That's because the tissue itself is corrugated, formed into tiny fingerlike projections covered with tentacles called villi. The villi snatch food as it drifts by, in much the same way that coral feeds on floating plankton. The villi absorb the nutritional molecules into the intestinal wall, where they pass into the blood and lymph systems and from there to every cell in the body that needs them. What isn't absorbed passes down into the colon in liquid form—the walls of the colon are like a giant sponge that sends most of the water back into the body. And in the colon, as we described in the first chapter, the undigested fiber is grabbed up by the bacteria who live there who ferment it into protective compounds called short-chain fatty acids. Finally, the waste products are sent packing, making the passage through the last piece of GI tract tubing, the sigmoid colon, before being pooped out of the body.

The "How" of Eating

While the digestive system might seem like its own self-contained world, the way we think about food and how we actually eat it set the tone for the entire enterprise. As we said, the anticipation of eating stimulates the enzymes in our saliva. But it also primes the digestive pump throughout the whole GI tract. The body actually secretes digestive enzymes and hydrochloric acid needed for proper digestion *before* you've swallowed a mouthful of food. If we eat without tuning in to our hunger or the pleasure we get from satisfying it—in other words, if the salivary enzymes aren't flowing and we're gulping instead of taking the time to chew thoroughly— the food won't be sufficiently broken down at the beginning of the trip and it won't be completely absorbed in the small intestine. Instead, it will become food for the bacteria that live there, leading to a condition you may have heard of called SIBO (small intestinal bacterial overgrowth) and the digestive upset and inflammation it can cause. Whereas we want to feed the friendly bacteria in our colon—it's one of the key nutritional messages of this book—we don't want to overfeed the much smaller number that hang out in our small intestine. Likewise, if we overfeed the unfriendly bacteria in the colon with a poor diet, those now more populous bugs can travel back up into the small intestine, where they can cause more trouble.

Using the mind to eat in tune with your digestive system means remembering a few simple things about *how* to eat. Anticipate the meal to come. Chew slowly. No one has derived a scientifically valid formula here (there is such a thing as being *too* meticulous), but Dr. Klaus Bielefeldt, director of the Neurogastroenterology and Motility Center at the University of Pittsburgh, says about ten chews per bite is in the ballpark. Take moderate-size forkfuls of food—you know when you're overloading—and put down the fork between bites. By slowing down the eating process moderately (you don't have to wait so long that your food gets cold), you're giving the body a chance to catch up. It takes about twenty to thirty minutes for stretch receptors in the stomach and hormones produced in the gut to signal the brain that the stomach has expanded and that the body's need for energy has been met. The brain interprets this as "fullness," or at least not being hungry anymore. If you gulp, you miss the memo and eat more than you need or really want. This brings with it a host of consequences, starting with too many calories, which drives weight gain, or, at a minimum, blocks weight loss. It also reduces the amount of empty space in the stomach that it needs to efficiently smash the food into smaller, easier-to-digest particles. Both too much food and too little space can contribute to less-than-optimal digestion and an irritable bowel!

HARA HACHI BU

This practice comes from the Okinawan culture and it means, simply, eating until you are 80 percent full. Words to live by. Stop eating when you are no longer hungry. The point of a good meal is not to keep eating until you feel uncomfortably distended. You may need some mindful eating practice to find your *hara hachi bu* "bliss spot." (See the sidebar on page 45.)

The "When" of Eating

Over the past decade or so, a lot of nutritionists and doctors latched on to the idea that "grazing," spreading five or six smaller meals over the course of the day, was a healthier and more weight-loss-friendly way to eat. The logic made sense—the smaller meals would keep blood sugar and insulin levels steadier—it just turned out not to be in sync with how the body wants to work. When we eat, the food doesn't drop through the GI tract through force of gravity. It's propelled down on waves of muscular contraction generated by the muscles of the gut wall. What scientists have more recently come to understand is that when we *don't* eat, the body takes advantage of the fasting state to generate a similar wave of contraction to clear out any remaining food particles in the upper GI tract and send it down to the colon, where it can be processed and disposed of. The whole process takes about ninety minutes. The scientists call this gut self-cleaning feature the "migrating motor complex," or in plain English, "the cleansing wave of the gut." When the gut doesn't get the necessary downtime between meals, once again, the risk is bacterial overgrowth in the small intestine and the gas, bloat and pain that often ensue.

I encourage my clients to observe a "sacred space" after a meal—some nutritionists prefer the more prosaic "rest and digest." Does this translate into your mother's or grandmother's admonition to eat "three squares"? Pretty much, except that in today's extended workday corporate culture, the time gap between lunch and dinner can grow well beyond the four-hour mark that usually spells hunger. A recent British survey of a thousand people who had resolved to watch their weight found that almost half had fallen off the wagon in the late afternoon, the average time of straying, 4:12 P.M.! So a healthy late-afternoon snack can be an excellent idea, a piece of fruit or modest-sized serving of nuts.

What's important is that most of our days have a predictable rhythm that suits the innate clock that's built into our physiology. Researchers now talk about "clock genes" distributed throughout the cells of our body that respond, for instance, to light and dark. (I'll talk more about this in the final MENDS chapter, Chapter 6, "S: Sustaining Practices.") Taking pleasure in meals at set times of the day is an important ritual that helps regulate that internal clock and gives the day its satisfying rhythm.

The Second Brain

From my brief description of the digestive tract, you now have some idea of how elaborate the system really is. Everything has to work just so. Hunger at the right time triggers the consumption of the right amount of food to be broken down by the right amount of digestive secretions. In fact, it's such a big job that over time, we evolved a gut with a mind of its own, a "second brain" that handled the mechanics of digestion in concert with the brain in our heads, but below the level of conscious awareness . . . as long as everything works the way it should. When it doesn't, we're all too aware of nausea, indigestion, constipation, diarrhea and the rest.

For the past thirty years or so, science has filled in the amazing details about the gut's enteric nervous system, housed mostly in the small intestine. It contains as many neurons as the spinal cord and it produces all of the same chemicals as the brain—dopamine, GABA (gamma-aminobutyric acid), acetylcholine and 95 percent of the body's supply of the feel-good neurotransmitter serotonin. The central highway that these chemicals travel, linking brain and gut, is the vagus nerve, which stretches from the base of the brain to the middle of the colon. The gut tells the brain how digestion is coming along—how full the stomach is, for example—and the brain responds accordingly, increasing or decreasing hunger. And the stress hormones that are orchestrated by the brain travel a similar path, which is why we can have those "gut-wrenching" experiences. The brain responds to threats or challenges in the outside world and the gut feels, well, a kick in the gut. In fact, stress often triggers digestive problems and it's certainly a major contributor to unwanted weight gain. High cortisol levels pump up the body's production of insulin and too much insulin directs the body to store calories as fat instead of burning them for energy.

The microbiome revolution of the past few years has made it clear that the "gut-brain axis" is a two-way street. And the gut isn't just sending progress reports on the mechanics of digestion. The gut bacteria are directly affecting how we think and feel, often about things that have nothing to do with digestion. Consider a mouse experiment done by a leading researcher, Stephen Collins, at Canada's McMaster University. He transferred gut bacteria from a group of gregarious mice into a group of timid, fearful mice who, lo and behold, became much bolder. In another experiment, rat pups that had high levels of stress hormones after being separated from their mothers calmed down after being fed a probiotic bacteria commonly found in yogurt. Collins's conclusion: the gut bacteria were "influencing behavior on a real-time basis." Other studies have shown that these probiotic strains altered the rodents' production of the neurotransmitter GABA in ways that mimic the effect of human antidepressant drugs. "These bacteria are, in effect, mind-altering microorganisms," says Mark Lyte at Texas Tech University, another researcher in the field. Science is adding a whole new dimension to the old line, "You are what you eat."

Yes, these are only animal studies. But these experiments provide us with clues to make sense of an extensive human research literature that shows that mental health and gut health are intimately connected. For instance, depression often shows up in people who first develop gut disorders. As UCLA researcher Kristin Tillisch put it, "Time and time again, we hear from patients that they never felt depressed or anxious until they started experiencing problems with their gut." Last year, Dr. Tillisch published a proof-of-concept study that showed you could change the way a person's brain worked by influencing the composition of the bacteria in the gut just slightly. Her study looked at eating a probiotic yogurt twice a day for four weeks. The women who ate the yogurt saw changes in the way their brains lit up on a functional magnetic resonance imaging scan (fMRI) compared to the women who did not. There were subtle differences in the way the brains processed sensory information and emotion.

On the weight front, Dr. Blaser at NYU has discovered that American kids, living in a relatively hygienic environment and regularly dosed with antibiotics, often lack a particular type of bacteria that humans have harbored in the stomach for millennia. This bacteria looks to keep in check the hormone ghrelin, which triggers the feeling of hunger in the brain. Lose the bacteria, it seems, and you lose a brake on appetite. How big a role this might play in the obesity epidemic of the past several decades, at this point, we can only guess.

Here's what we do know about the "cross talk" between brain and

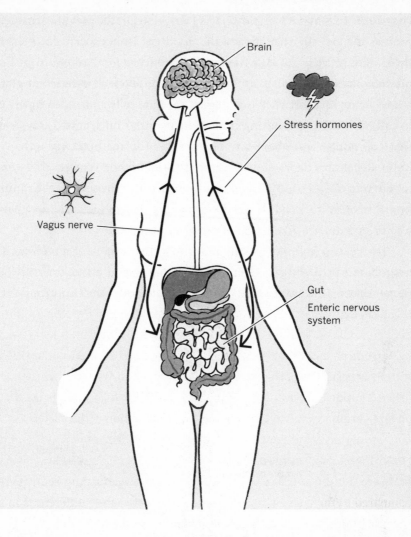

microbiota. Stress hormones, controlled by the brain, can directly change how the bacteria in the gut affect the gut's production of hormones and neurochemicals that speak to the brain, including the ones that affect appetite. And stress hormones, by changing the conditions inside the gut—for instance, the amount of mucus produced to line the gut wall—can favor certain bacterial strains over others, again affecting the chemical messengers that drive the enteric nervous system. The stress hormones may also increase the permeability of the gut wall, making it leakier and allowing fragments of bad bacteria to escape into the bloodstream, triggering a systemic inflammatory response. (As I described in the previous chapter, a processed-food diet that starves the good gut bacteria can do the same thing.) Or, in their guise as the immune system's forward guard, the gut microbiota may respond to unfamiliar bacteria or a food irritant like gluten as an enemy invader. They may signal immune cells embedded in the gut to call out the troops, setting in motion a similar inflammatory response that can impact just about any organ system in the body, including the brain. Recall that depression and anxiety are common symptoms of gluten intolerance. Depression in turn saps people of the energy and the motivation they need to make smart food choices and to exercise, driving up weight gain and the likelihood of digestive problems.

The central highway joining brain to gut? It's more of a beltway. The microbiome is directly linked to the immune system, the endocrine (hormone) system, the brain and its stress response, even the skin. Everything is connected!

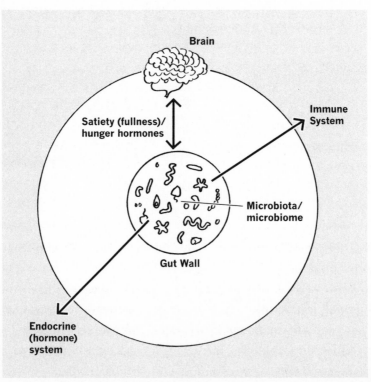

Mindful Eating

That was a lot to digest, wasn't it? I've noticed when I present some of this material at my digestive health workshops, the students may find the science interesting (some may not), but what they really get excited about are the techniques we teach them to lower their stress levels and increase their emotional resiliency. That is, after all, the most powerful way to get your brain and your gut back on good speaking terms.

I'll go into some detail on mind-body exercises that cool down the stress response and focus awareness in Chapter 6. But let's set the stage right now with this simple, everyday technique.

BELLY BREATHING

Try this for five minutes every day and shed some energy-draining stress. Find a comfortable chair or cushion and sit, relaxed but upright, eyes open or closed, as you like. Release the tension in your shoulders and let them drop comfortably. For the next several minutes, take steady deep breaths in whatever way feels most natural to you. You may notice that as your breathing grows more relaxed, you are breathing more from the diaphragm (you can see your belly push out on the inhales) and less from the chest. The air reaches to the bottom of your lungs, stimulating the vagus nerve and triggering the body's relaxation response, slowing heart rate and lowering blood pressure. Feel the coolness of the inhalation, the warmth of the exhalation.

Now let's consider this calm state of being in the context of your relationship with food.

Over the past decade, an entire therapeutic movement has grown up around "mindful eating," complete with supporting organizations like the Center for Mind-Body Medicine (cmbm.org) and the Center for Mindful Eating (thecenterformindfuleating.org). It addresses the challenges of food cravings and "emotional eating" from a Buddhist-influenced perspective that emphasizes the importance of quieting the mind and being "in the moment." (When you do the belly-breathing exercise, notice, if you really relax into it, that the usual internal mental chatter quiets down.) It makes so much sense! For a lot of women with weight and digestive issues, food comes to represent so much more than a tasty or a nutritious meal. It becomes a lot of things: a test of willpower, a reminder of past humiliations, a prompt for a host of sad or happy memories.

Think about my client Anna and all the anxieties that commonly attach to our effort to gain control over food. The mindfulness approach encourages you to focus your attention on the food in front of you, "peace in the present moment." You learn with practice to nourish your body when there is physical hunger, not when your mind is craving some sort of emotional release. There's a huge behavioral science literature that shows that people who are attuned to their body's hunger signals are more successful at managing their weight than people whose eating habits are more influenced by external cues, whether that's a TV advertisement or what their friend just ordered at a restaurant or some fixed idea about what they should or shouldn't be doing to lose weight. For many of us, tuning in to our bodies and eating mindfully take practice. It *is* a practice.

Here's the advice that neuroscientist Sandra Aamodt gave at a high-profile TED (Technology, Entertainment, Design) conference last year: "Sit down to regular meals without distractions. Think about how your body feels when you start to eat and when you stop and let your hunger decide when you should be done." Does that sound *too* simple? Dr. Aamodt says she struggled with weight and self-esteem issues her entire life. When she finally understood that food wasn't a means to assert her self-worth, that it was food, nothing more, nothing less, the neurosis dropped away.

If people like Anna and Sandra Aamodt used to invest food with too much meaning, many of my clients don't pay enough attention to it. They're "mindless" eaters, snacking on whatever's at hand over the course of the day. For people in both camps, the mindfulness prescription that focuses on the sensory experience of eating can reform counterproductive habits. In a pilot study done by researchers at the University of San Francisco, the obese women in a group of overweight women who trained in mindful eating and meditation for four months lowered their cortisol levels and maintained their body weight. Their counterparts who received no training had no change in their elevated cortisol levels and gained weight.

In my workshops, I might spend fifteen minutes getting my students to really taste a grape. First, they'll just look at it and be aware of the saliva forming in their mouths, the initial wave of "cephalic" digestion. They'll put it in their mouths and sit with it there for maybe a minute. One woman told me recently that she'd never before been aware of the texture of a grape skin. Then they'll chew it slowly, becoming attuned to its specific grapey sweetness, even the sound of it in their mouths. At my last workshop, another woman said she found this simple exercise to be a "sensual experience." They were really alive to the moment!

Obviously, this isn't something you're likely to do at home every day. But here's a practice that you can do at any meal. It puts you in touch with slower eating, which is good for digestion and appetite control (those satiety hormones have time to kick in), and with the food itself.

EATING: A SENSUAL EXERCISE

Take three relaxing breaths.

Engage your senses:

Think about your food.

Eyes (look at your food)

Nose (take in the aromas)

Mouth (chew your food thoroughly)

Rest your hands in your lap every few bites and breathe again.

The Emotional and Spiritual Wisdom of Weight Loss

As useful, even liberating, as the new microbiome science is, the weight-loss and digestive-health journey can't just be boiled down to gut bacteria, satiety hormones and high-fiber foods. There's a rich emotional and even spiritual dimension to this landscape. How could there not be? You're breaking out of old habits and routines, testing yourself in new situations and, let's be honest, risking failure. You're confronting the idea of hunger and engaging anxieties and hopes about your physical appearance and your health.

I've worked with clients whose eating is fueled by loneliness, by stress, by boredom, by habit. This list is hardly exhaustive—I'm sure you can add a few more. But the common denominator is that these women were not feeling adequately *nourished* in some important aspect of their lives and they turned to food to make up the difference.

VISUALIZATION PRACTICE

Close your eyes and think about hunger. What makes you hungry? What do you crave? Is your appetite for food really the driving force here? Or is it standing in for some other not-entirely-satisfied hungers in your life, for love, respect, companionship? Whatever comes up, write it in a journal and revisit it over the next few days and weeks.

I have a client, Emma, a Harvard undergrad, with both digestive health and weight issues. She'd been obsessed with the extra fifteen pounds that she was carrying, and she got lost in self-blame and doubt. For her, something as simple as a "daily affirmation" has worked wonders. We were consulting on Skype and I said, "Emma, I want you to create a positive statement about all the changes you've made in your diet." And she said to me, "Well, eating this way helps me to feel my best." It gave me chills to hear her say that. I could hear that those simple words had such meaning for her. I told her, "Every time you go to a dark place or you get upset by a number on the scale, repeat those words: 'Eating this way helps me to feel my best.'" We had created a daily affirmation for her, an easy way for her to call on her internal sources of self-calming and support. I am convinced that the weight came off in large part because of this reframing affirmation.

AFFIRMATION OF THE BREATH

Repeat this to yourself as often as you like, daily or whenever you're feeling stressed or less in control than you'd like to be: "My breath is my source of calm." Try coming up with another affirmation that speaks to the circumstances of your life and that, when you concentrate and say it to yourself over and over again, has a calming and reassuring effect.

In the book *Zen Mind, Beginner's Mind*, which introduced so many Westerners to Zen, Shunryu Suzuki wrote, "The beginner's mind is the mind of compassion." That's the mind that I'd like you to leave this first MENDS chapter with: bighearted and open-minded, without false optimism or self-defeating despair. False optimism is the currency of most diets and weight-loss books that push the idea that all you need to do to lose weight is to cut back calories for a while and to cycle through different foods on some kind of regimen; in other words, ignore the hunger and you're home free. Despair enters the picture when this approach predictably fails, over and over again, and you convince yourself you must be lacking some essential quality required for success.

In our culture, women tend to be hard on themselves, often putting everyone else first and ignoring their own needs. There's this pressure to be perfect. And perfect is the enemy of self-compassion, of self-forgiveness. That's why I love the Eastern concept of practice. We don't have to succeed at a practice; we just have to keep doing it, and if we do, we get better at it. Our resolve is not to be perfect on a diet. Instead, we commit to a practice of healthy eating and living that, even with the inevitable slipups, deepens and ripens with time. May MENDS be your guide to true nourishment.

THE INTENTION CARD

Take an index card or some other small, more attractive card and write, in just a few sentences, why you are committed to losing weight and keeping it off. It could be anything from needing to stay healthy so you can play with your children or grandchildren to wanting to fit into those size 6 or size 8 dresses in your closet. Don't worry if your motivation sounds virtuous or not—if it's important to you, it's important! Put the card in your purse or wallet, and in moments when you feel your resolve slipping, take it out and read it again. Stay connected to your intention and your intuition.

LOVE LETTER

In a spirit of self-acceptance, write a short love letter to your body. Then have your body write a love letter to you. Express whatever feelings you have for your body, good or perhaps not so good. You may discover that it's the first time in memory that you've looked at your physical self with a less than critical eye. I've had clients write things like, "My weight isn't where I'd like it to be or my gut's a mess, but I've got good bone structure or my eyes are lovely." They forgive their bodies and they forgive themselves for not having paid enough attention to their health and well-being. Sometimes the body will write back something like: "I'm here for you. We're going to accept this new challenge together."

Chapter 3

E: ELIMINATE THE "PROBLEM" FOODS

Susan

Susan is a professional photographer and a single mom who for most of her adult life had suffered from IBS-type symptoms—bloating, diarrhea, constipation—as well as reflux/heartburn. Hard-to-shed extra weight was an issue as well. When she moved to the Berkshires region two years ago and began to pay more attention to her diet, taking advantage of the fresh produce and fruit in the warmer months, she figured she'd start seeing and feeling some positive results. Instead, she got worse. In addition to her old problems, she felt continually dragged out, with no energy to spare, and she would break out in nasty eczema rashes on a regular basis. She often felt anxious, which was strange since she always had thought of herself as an adventurous, artistic sort of person. Finally, an Internet search of her symptoms turned up a clue, a possible sensitivity to gluten. A lightbulb went on in her head. Since moving to the area, she'd discovered a local bakery and its fresh whole-wheat bread, which she thought was healthy as long as she didn't overindulge. But Susan's self-diagnosis was tossed out the window by her local physician when she didn't test positive for celiac disease, the severe form of gluten intolerance. (He gave her an ointment for the eczema and suggested an antidepressant for her low energy and anxiety.) Thankfully, Susan came across my book on digestive health, The Inside Tract, *in a local bookstore and sought me out. Together, we came up with a weight-loss and digestive-health "elimination diet" that excluded gluten and most dairy products. (It was identical to Weeks 1 and 2 of the Swift Plan in Chapter 7.) After a month, we carefully reintroduced these foods and discovered that, yes, indeed, her reaction to gluten had caused the inflammation that was at the root of her problems. Without the gluten, her whole foods–based diet produced the positive changes in her weight and digestion that she'd expected all along. The skin, energy and anxiety issues all resolved over time. Even the reflux improved. She felt like herself again.*

SELF-INQUIRY BOX

1. Have you noticed that "healthy" foods like whole-wheat bread sometimes leave you feeling anything but good?
2. Have you noticed that if you eat too much high-fiber plant foods, such as cauliflower or black beans, you can trigger an upset gut?
3. Do half or more of your daily calories come from processed foods?

'm not a naysayer by temperament. If I had a choice, I'd much rather talk about the fabulous things that the right foods can do for your health and weight than what the wrong ones can do to derail it. But as a nutritionist, I appreciate that diet is a two-part proposition. You need to eliminate, or aggressively cut back, the problem foods to give your metabolism and your digestion the window they need to recover. That is the E, for "eliminate," in MENDS. At the same time, you introduce or increase the foods that build up your resilience and protect against disease while fueling a leaner, cleaner metabolism. That's a story for the next chapter, "N: Nourish the Body, and the Belly."

Susan's story illustrates one way the wrong food can make the gut, and life, miserable. She has a sensitivity to a food component, a protein compound called gluten, found in wheat and most of the grain products we commonly eat. As you may remember from the first chapter, the microbiome serves as the immune system's first line of defense in the gut. If the bacteria don't recognize a food compound passing through the gut as a friend, they signal to the immune cells embedded in the gut wall to respond to this foreigner. The result is, you guessed it, inflammation, which can disturb the gut (Susan's IBS-type symptoms) and create problems virtually anywhere in the body (her fatigue and skin issues).

The solution to Susan's case, and to the cases of hundreds if not thousands of my clients, is to identify the food that's triggering the problem and get rid of it. In this chapter, I've pulled together a master list of potentially troubling foods that can upset digestion and weight control that, one way or another, work through the gut and the bacteria that live there—the MicroMenaces.

But as you'll also remember from Chapter 1, the microbiome can set in motion digestion and weight problems in another, more under-the-radar way. (There was nothing subtle about Susan's reaction to gluten—she was wiped out.) We're not dealing with specific gut irritants here but rather with an overall imbalance in the foods we choose and the quantities in which we eat them. If we eat the wrong foods in the wrong amounts, we'll wind up feeding the bacteria that can do us harm at the expense of the bacteria that help us. This is a different pathway than the food sensitivity that plagued Susan, but it leads to the same result—chronic, low-grade systemic inflammation that promotes an unhappy gut, weight gain and, again, symptoms that can show up anywhere in the body.

How does a food choice turn into a MicroMenace? As we go down the list, three big, and overlapping, reasons will jump out:

1. Not enough fiber to properly feed the microbiome.
2. Too many nutrient-poor calories, promoting inflammatory weight gain.
3. A specific food or food ingredient, like gluten, that upsets the digestive system or triggers systemic inflammation or both.

MicroMenaces

#1 "Dense" Carbs

For years, nutritionists and popular diet books have been chasing the holy grail of the perfect diet, that just-right ratio of carbs to protein to fat. But finally there is a scientific consensus that dovetails with what I've always practiced—the exact percentages of calories are much less important than the quality of those calories. And yes, the total number of calories you are consuming does matter. (If you're eating plant-based foods in the portions I recommend, you don't have to count calories. It's what some nutritionists call a "non-diet approach to eating.") In fact, when medical anthropologists looked at the diets of indigenous peoples around the globe, they discovered that some had a diet high in carbs (root vegetables and fruit), some had a diet high in fats (nuts and some meat) and it didn't seem to make any difference. What these traditional peoples had in common was that they weren't overweight and they didn't suffer from the diet-related diseases of aging that ultimately drag most of us down—heart disease, type 2 diabetes, obesity.

So what are today's remaining hunter-gatherers, and our Paleo ancestors, doing right that we've got so wrong? As Ian Spreadbury, a brilliant scientist at Canada's Queen's University, pointed out in a recent influential paper, the biggest difference looks to be that the hunter-gatherers consume their carbs, the body's primary energy source, in the form of seeds and plants and fruits. We moderns grind up the seeds into grain flour and create concentrated sugars from what's naturally found in sugarcane, beets and corn. In the process, we've lost most of the fiber and concentrated the calories in fast-digesting food bombs.

Spreadbury calls these carbs "acellular" because the cell walls of the plants have been broken down by this processing before we cook it or eat it. As a result, they are quickly digested and absorbed by the body, driving up blood sugar and insulin, which, as we discussed in the first chapter, can fuel systemic inflammation and weight gain. Spreadbury has captured this idea in a measure he calls "carbohydrate density," similar to "glycemic load," which you may have heard of (see the sidebar below.)

TAKING THE MEASURE OF FOOD

Carbohydrate density is a measure of the amount of carbohydrate in 100 grams of a particular food. Sugar, flour, and refined grain products have a high carb density! This measure is emerging as an important way to determine whether a food promotes inflammation and obesity.

Glycemic index (GI) is a measure of how quickly blood glucose (sugar) rises after eating a particular type of food. Technically speaking, it estimates how much each gram of available carbohydrate (total carbohydrate minus fiber) in a food raises a person's blood glucose level after being eaten, as compared with the consumption of pure glucose, which has a GI of 100.

Glycemic load (GL) is derived from the glycemic index (GI). It's widely considered a more useful measure than GI, since it takes into account the actual carbohydrate content of the food, while GI does not. Some fruits—watermelon, for example—have a high GI but a low GL. The lower the GL, the better!

Let's bring this down to earth. The brown-rice cake seems so virtuous because it only has 70 calories, but most of those calories are carbohydrate, so the carb density is actually pretty high. A medium-sized sweet potato is about 100 calories and it too is carb-rich, but because it's loaded with fiber and water, the carb density is considerably lower. *Low carb density is better—* it will take longer to break down to sugar in the bloodstream. Some popular diets ban fruit because it contains a fair amount of sugar. But even pineapple, the poster child for high-glycemic fruit, has a lower carb density than a brown-rice cake because it's packed with fiber and water.

Now we can make sense of an important 2011 Harvard study that found that high levels of consumption of certain types of food, like potato chips and French fries, was an excellent predictor of weight gain over time. The junk-food crowd was gorging on the "dense carbs" and it showed on their waistlines.

So when I place dense carbs number 1 on my MicroMenace list, I'm *not* demonizing all carbohydrates. As I'll detail in the next chapter, the non-starchy vegetables that are the cornerstone of the Swift Diet are made up of fiber-rich carbohydrate (that and a lot of water). It's the processed-food dense carbs, the quick-to-digest carbs, that we need to eliminate. I think most of us have accepted the fact that a cookie, or refined-grain cereals with a ton of added sugar, is not the acme of healthy eating, for the microbiome or for any other system in the body. But what about whole-wheat grains, let's say the tasty multigrain bread you buy at the supermarket or the health food store? True, the fibrous plant germ (the plant embryo) and the bran (the seed coat) are added to the flour so it's a better choice than a loaf of fluffy white Wonder Bread. But the flour itself is, to use Spreadbury's language, "acellular"; these dense carbs are quick to be digested and absorbed by the body.

> **Swift Bottom Line:** Whole foods like vegetables, fruits and legumes that have their cell walls intact are "smart carbs" with a low carb density. You don't need to have a carb density or GL/GI calculator by your plate; just avoid the processed, refined carbs. Carbohydrate consciousness that considers both quality (low carb density) and quantity (neither too little nor too much carb) is the first step on the path to healthy weight!

The Insulin Connection

Of the three macronutrients that make up our diet—carbs, fat, protein— only carbohydrate significantly stimulates the body's production of insulin, the hormone that escorts the sugar from the blood into the cells of the body, to be burned for energy or stored as fat. Both protein and fat can be burned for energy, but they have different primary jobs. The body uses protein to build the cells that provide structure (organs, muscle, bones) and the cells (enzymes, hormones and so on) that direct the whole show. Fat is the raw material for cell membranes and certain types of hormones.

For most people, the single biggest "bang for the buck" they get when they reform their diet is replacing dense carbs with smart carbs. Another way of putting this is: replacing processed, refined carbs with the fiber-rich, unrefined version. In one fell swoop, they decrease the calories that they're taking in and reduce the amount of insulin the body has to produce to convert those calories into energy. The net result: a more effective calorie burn with fewer calories going into the fat storage locker. One Harvard study analyzed the diets of nearly two thousand Costa Ricans and found that merely substituting one serving of beans for one serving of white rice a day dropped the risk of developing metabolic syndrome (prediabetes) by 35 percent.

Remember the traditional explanation for weight gain: more calories coming into the system than being burned (calories in/calories out). It turns out that dense carbs promote weight gain by affecting how efficiently we burn calories as well (calories out). In 2012, my friend Dr. David Ludwig, at Boston Children's Hospital, published an elegant study in *The Journal of the American Medical Association* that looked at three groups of people after they'd lost 10 to 15 percent of their body weight in the first part of the study. He rotated the groups through three different diets that all had the same number of calories. The group that ate the conventionally healthy diet, with lots of whole-grain carbs, burned fewer calories a day than either the group whose low-glycemic carbs came mostly from legumes and veggies, or the group on the low-carb diet with lots of protein and fat. (The last group actually had the best numbers, but Dr. Ludwig had health concerns about going so low on the carbs, which in practice means a lot more protein and fat in the diet. I'll delve into that shortly.) These results suggest that people who rely on grains as a dietary mainstay, even whole grains, are at greater risk for regaining the pounds after they've lost weight, which, sad to say, is what happens to most people.

The public health establishment is slowly getting the message. The USDA's 2011 My Plate dietary advice recommends a daily diet of over

30 percent grains, still too high if you're striving for healthy gut and weight. But compare that to the government's 1992 Food Pyramid. The bottom, largest block of the pyramid was grains, any kind of grains, with a recommendation of six to eleven servings of bread, cereal, pasta and rice a day!

(Microscopic) Gut Check

Let's check in on what's going on at the microscopic level. When we eat a diet heavy with dense carbs, we're overfeeding the small intestine, where the sugars are broken down and absorbed into the bloodstream through the wall of the small intestine. Too much sugar, too fast and, as we said, we're setting the table for insulin surges, supersized sweet cravings and weight gain. But that's only half the story. The other half is what we're *not* eating, the fiber-rich plant foods that feed the bacteria in the colon. "It's starvation in the midst of plenty," is how University of Pittsburgh gastroenterologist Stephen O'Keefe puts it. As we mentioned in the first chapter, if our friends in the gut, the bifidobacteria and lactobacilli, don't get enough to eat, they decline in number and can't ferment enough organic acids to properly maintain the lining of the gut that keeps the messy business of digestion walled off from the rest of the body. (One leading microbiome researcher, Justin Sonnenburg, at Stanford, discovered that the friendly bacteria can get so hungry, they'll resort to eating the gut lining itself!) Because less organic acid is being produced, the pH balance of the gut changes and becomes more hospitable to opportunistic troublemakers such as unfriendly bacteria and fungi. Bits and pieces of them slip through the now depleted gut wall into the bloodstream and provoke a system-wide inflammation. This can cause insulin resistance and weight gain as well as enervating symptoms like fatigue and brain fog.

Leaky gut is probably the best-studied type of MicroObesity, but scientists are looking at a number of ways that gut bacteria can influence weight. It's been discovered, for instance, that certain types of bacteria can extract more calories more efficiently from a given amount of food. People who harbor greater numbers of these bugs are thought to be vulnerable to becoming overweight.

Paleo Perspective

Researchers like Leach and Sonnenburg are telling us that the more energy we can get from bacteria breaking down fiber in the colon and fermenting it, the more our gut will resemble that of today's hunter-gatherers (and yesterday's Paleo Woman) and the better off we'll be. Paleo scientists estimate that our ancestors ate at least 70 grams of fiber a day, significantly more than the current government dietary recommendation, and got about 30 percent of their calories from fermentation in the gut. And we know from studies of surviving hunter-gatherer tribes that their digestive systems aren't generating the kind of inflammation, and health and weight problems, that accompany today's highly refined convenience-driven diet. Take your pick, SAD (Standard American Diet) or MAD (Modern American Diet)! To take one example from the research literature, Dr. O'Keefe authored a study that linked the rich diversity of gut bacteria in subjects from rural Africa, where colon cancer is relatively rare, with the lower bacterial diversity in a matched group of African Americans with much higher colon cancer rates.

Now at this point you may be wondering about the Paleo Diet, which, in its various incarnations, has generated a lot of interest and book sales. The Paleo Diet has yet to be rigorously researched, but in a few small clinical studies it's yielded some nice results, dropping waist circumference and lowering heart disease risk. In theory, I'm all for it. But in practice, a lot of modern Paleo proponents recommend mega meat portions. Because today's Paleos tend not to be as creative foragers as their ancient forebearers, they often rely on a lot of animal protein to make up the caloric shortfall that comes with eliminating grains. A few years ago, two leading researchers who had helped put the Paleo Diet on the map revised their thinking and concluded that a true Paleo pyramid would be built on a foundation of vegetables and fruit, not meat. And as I'll discuss in a minute, too much meat can contribute to gut and overall health problems. The Swift Diet takes a flexitarian approach: plenty of plant foods with limited amounts of animal protein and whole grains like quinoa and buckwheat, providing a nice variety in taste, texture and nutrition. You might be interested to know that the most recent anthropological detective work has uncovered the fact that the original Paleo people did themselves eat a limited amount of legumes and grains. They ground up wild grasses mortar-and-pestle style.

A Matter of Timing

When you get down to it, the problem with dense carbs is timing. Our grain-based agriculture is only about ten thousand years old. That's not an issue for the microbiota, which adapts to whatever it's being fed in a matter of days. It *is* a problem for our human metabolism, which evolved over hundreds of thousands of years on a fiber-rich diet without developing the systems to handle the fallout from whole-wheat bagels and Lean Cuisines. Maybe in another ten thousand years it will. In the meantime, we need to make some dietary changes to protect our health and shed the excess weight, starting with cutting out the highly processed dense carbs.

#2 Sugar: The Not-So-Sweet Truth

Sugar is the ultimate dense carb. It's a pure hit of food energy to the system, quickly absorbed by the body, unlike more complex starches that are broken down more slowly before they can be absorbed. The result is metabolic chaos:

- Sugar depletes your energy level
- Sugar stimulates cravings for more sugar and sweet stuff
- Sugar impairs your immune system
- Sugar feeds your stress hormones
- Sugar drives fat storage
- Sugar raises your cholesterol and triglycerides
- Sugar disturbs insulin regulation
- Sugar disrupts digestive health

And the stuff is ubiquitous. Sugar, both ordinary table sugar (sucrose) and a supersweet industrial version, high-fructose corn syrup, finds its way into almost every morsel of processed food in this country, which, per person, breaks down to forty-seven pounds of fructose consumed annually, forty pounds of table sugar. We eat, on average, twenty-two teaspoons of added sugar a day! And clearly, added sugar must be undermining metabolism in a number of ways. It's been linked to high blood pressure, increase in fats in the blood and insulin resistance. In a February 2014 study published in *JAMA Internal Medicine*, Harvard researchers calculated that people who consumed more than 21 percent of their daily calories from added sugar doubled the risk of dying from heart disease compared to those who got less than 10 percent of their calories that way. And yet, as a society, we keep gorging. That same study estimated that Americans as a group get 15 percent of their daily calories from added sugar.

SUGAR SMARTS

1. Learn the language. The chemical ID for most sugars has an "ose" ending, including: dextrose, galactose, glucose, fructose, lactose, maltose, mannose, sucrose.
2. Seek and you will find the Fifty Shades of Sugar. To identify hidden sugar on a food label, you need to become familiar with the obvious and some of the not-so-obvious aliases that also mean sugar: agave nectar, barley malt, beet sugar, blackstrap molasses, brown sugar, cane juice, cane sugar, caramel, carob syrup, castor sugar, coconut sugar, confectioners' sugar, corn syrup, date sugar, demerara sugar, dextrin, evaporated cane juice, fructose, fruit juice concentrate, glucose syrup, high-fructose corn syrup (HFCS), honey, invert sugar, malt syrup, maltodextrin, maple syrup, molasses, raw sugar, rice syrup, syrup, treacle, and turbinado sugar.
3. Translate the numbers. Look for the total grams of sugar per serving and convert to teaspoons so you better understand the sugar load. The cold hard facts: every 4 grams of sugar = 1 teaspoon. For example, 28 grams of sugar in a serving of cereal = 7 teaspoons!

4. Be a label sleuth. Sugar labeling is deceptive. For one thing, the Nutrition Facts do not differentiate between naturally occurring sugars and highly processed sugars that are added to the product. One example is plain, unsweetened yogurt, which comes in at about 15 grams sugar, but there is no added sugar. The grams of sugar come from the lactose, which is a natural part of the product. And although I recommend limiting total sugar load, start by eliminating the highly processed foods with their tsunami of added sugars.

5. Be cautious about sugar alcohols or polyols. These sweet additives often show up in "sugar-free" gums, candies, oral care products and medications and can be especially problematic for an irritable bowel. Here are a few of the more common ones: erythritol, glycerol, hydrogenated starch hydrolysate, isomalt, lactitol, maltitol, mannitol, polydextrose, sorbitol and xylitol.

6. Be sensible about herbal sweeteners such as stevia, Lo Han Guo, miracle fruit and countless others being promoted in the expanding sweetener marketplace. For example, stevia, although touted as a natural sweetener, delivers a sweet burst that is about three hundred times sweeter than sugar. Better to wean your taste buds off the supersweet than rely on processed herbal alternatives.

The Sweet Rush

These sour statistics on national sugar consumption highlight a mega-problem with this MicroMenace. It really can be highly addictive. Do you think that language is overblown? My friend Kelly Brownell, recently appointed a dean of public policy at Duke University, doesn't. He developed the well-known Yale Food Addiction Scale and compares an addiction to highly processed food to other potentially pathological attractions like sex and gambling (yaleruddcenter.org/resources/upload/docs/what/addiction/foodaddictionscale09.pdf). Dr. Robert Lustig, a University of California, San Francisco, endocrinologist who researches sugar's effect on the gut and the brain, says the government should regulate sugar the same way it does alcohol and tobacco. Both alcohol and sugar activate the same reward centers in the brain. In both cases, excess can be a disaster.

Whether it's the clients I work with privately or the students I teach in my workshops, the single biggest stumbling block is their craving for sweets. And yet I have plenty of clients who have fought a hard battle against weight their entire adult lives and after a week—*a week*—of clean eating and no added sugar, the craving loosens its grip. If you stop eating sugar-laden foods, the cravings will subside.

To get a better handle on the physiological reasons why people eat in ways that clearly don't serve their best interests, Dr. David Ludwig conducted an ingenious experiment, published in 2013. He fed milk shakes to a group of a dozen volunteers on two separate occasions using two different milk shake formulations. The study subjects thought they liked the milk shakes about the same, but their brains told a different story. Their brain scans showed more activation in the brain centers that regulate cravings and reward after drinking the milk shake with the higher-glycemic sweetener. This is in line with earlier studies that showed that the pleasure center in the brain lights up more brightly when a subject is presented with a slice of chocolate cake than when the food on offer is a plate of vegetables. This "sweet rush" tended to be greater in people who were overweight. And not surprisingly, the sweeter milk shake packed a metabolic wallop as well. Four hours after drinking it, the subjects' blood sugar levels had plummeted and they were hungrier than when they had drunk the lower-glycemic-index shake.

None of this should be surprising. For hundreds of thousands of years, we evolved as a species to seek out the relatively few sources of unprocessed sugar in nature—fruits, root vegetables and honey—as a nutritional hedge against starvation. Evolution has hardwired our sweet tooth. As the former FDA commissioner Dr. David Kessler described in *The End of Overeating*, and Pulitzer Prize–winning reporter Michael Moss amplified in *Salt Sugar Fat*, the food industry has exploited that vulnerability to sell us billions of dollars' worth of sucrose- and fructose-laden drinks, cookies and crackers.

Fructose and Sucrose: The Bitter Facts

Sugar in the form of fructose is found in some of the healthiest foods that nature provides: fruits, root vegetables, honey. In the body, fructose behaves differently than the other major sugar, glucose. When it's digested, it heads straight to the liver, without stimulating the production of insulin, usually a good thing. Really, the problem with fructose in nature is that it has the potential to upset the sensitive gut. Fructose is a card-carrying member of a group of carbohydrates that can feed the bacteria in our guts *too* well— we'll discuss this in detail later in this chapter. In the plant world, fructose is always partnered with glucose in fruits. But certain fruits, such as figs, apples and pears, are very high in fructose and relatively low in glucose. These are the ones that can over-ferment in the gut and aggravate IBS-type symptoms. We call this fructose intolerance or malabsorption.

But the major ugliness emerges when the fructose in corn is industrially converted to high-fructose corn syrup, or HFCS, and added to processed foods and drinks. In this concentrated, high-calorie form, stripped of the fiber that slows down digestion and the nutrients that enhance health, fructose does its dirty business. In the liver, it mostly gets converted into fat, raising cholesterol and triglyceride levels in the blood, a process scientists call lipogenesis. For some seventy million Americans, this hit to the liver contributes to fatty liver disease. In one small clinical study, the subjects who consumed the HFCS gained more belly fat than their counterparts who consumed the same amount of calories as glucose.

Research done by Dr. Lustig and Dr. Richard Johnson at the University of Colorado suggests that HFCS contributes to weight gain in another way. It gets in the way of leptin, a satiety hormone produced by our fat cells that tells our brain when we've had enough to eat. Other researchers argue that table sugar is just as good at confusing our hunger signals. Cold comfort. What is indisputable is that added sugars, fructose or sucrose, deliver a double whammy in soft drinks, sports drinks, and sweetened teas. Not only does the sugar promote leptin resistance, which blunts our ability to feel full, but liquid calories in any form aren't registered by the body as accurately as the calories in solid food. We don't compensate for them as effectively when it comes time to eat our next meal. And fruit juice, while it's more nutritious than a soft drink or a bottle of sweet tea, delivers a similar sugar hit. When fiber is removed from fruit to make fruit juice, you're left with a MicroMenace, so if you're going to drink fruit juice, I recommend a "nano-serving," not more than a couple of ounces, preferably diluted with water or seltzer. Take a look at the numbers. Between 1965 and 2002, when the percentage of Americans who were overweight and obese was skyrocketing, the percentage of daily calories we took in from beverages, mostly sugar-sweetened, almost doubled, from 11.8 percent to 21 percent.

I'm not asking you to be ashamed of your sweet tooth. It's how our ancestors survived. Honor it; build a shrine to it. But you can't negotiate with it. As you'll see, on the Swift Plan, processed foods with added sugars are out. They stimulate the appetite for more of the same and they coarsen our taste for naturally sweet foods. And so, for that matter, do low-calorie or no-calorie artificial sweeteners. First off, there is little good evidence that these fake-sugar compounds help with weight loss. In one 2013 study rats fed yogurt with either saccharin or aspartame gained more weight than their rodent counterparts who took their yogurt with simple table sugar.

ARRIVEDERCI ARTIFICIAL SWEETENERS!

Acesulfame-K (Sunett, Sweet & Safe, Sweet One)

Aspartame (Equal, NutraSweet)

Neotame or neohexyl-aspartame

Saccharin (Sweet'N Low)

Sucralose (Splenda)

Tagatose (Naturlose)

The fact that the number of Americans consuming artificial sweeteners more than doubled from 1987 to 2000, the same period of time when the national waistline was dramatically expanding, does not fill me with confidence that tricking the taste buds through chemistry is a good weight-loss strategy. Safety is probably the bigger issue. In one 2013 study, coauthored by a National Institutes of Health researcher, the popular artificial sweetener Splenda (sucralose) was found to release compounds that when heated are related to the infamous carcinogen dioxin! In rats, the stuff reduced the helpful bacteria in the gut, adding insult to injury!

The reeducation of the palette begins with what I call a Sweet Sabbatical. We replace the white menace with strong flavors provided by fruits and by herbs and spices, whether they're savory like rosemary and thyme or sweet tasting (but with precious few calories) like cinnamon and vanilla. Spiced Indian tea, chai, with no added sugar also makes for a soothing sweet alternative.

#3 Fats: Unfriendly and Too Much

The dietary fats story has changed radically since the days when doctors and diet gurus *knew* that dietary fat was the villain responsible for weight gain and heart disease. Yesterday's public enemy number one, saturated fat, has been rehabilitated, at least partially. And mass-produced vegetable oils like canola oil and corn oil, which until recently were considered healthy alternatives to saturated-fat-laden butter, are coming under increasing scrutiny.

The Fat Family

Let's rewind. Fatty acids, the building blocks of the fats we eat, come in three main types: monounsaturated, polyunsaturated and saturated. These terms refer to their chemical structure, how hydrogen is connected to the carbon chain in the fatty acid. But let's not get bogged down in biochemistry. For now, let's focus on when an oil change is in order; in the next chapter you will learn more about nourishment when it comes to the matter of fat!

- Monounsaturated fatty acids (MUFAs) are found abundantly in olives, olive oil, avocados, peanuts and most nuts and seeds and the oils made from them.
- Polyunsaturated fatty acids (PUFAs) are present in a wide range of plant foods as well as in fish that eat plants (algae). Two families of these polyunsaturated fats, the omega-3s and omega-6s, are considered "essential" fatty acids because our body doesn't make them, so we have to get them from our diet. (Thumbs-down to mass-produced omega-6-heavy vegetable oils.)
- Saturated fatty acids (SFAs) are found in high concentrations in animal foods—for example, dairy and meat—as well as in tropical oils like coconut, palm and palm kernel oil.
- Trans-fatty acids (TFAs) are naturally found in small amounts in some animal foods and in huge amounts in the processed-food supply, in "partially hydrogenated" oils like corn oil and soybean oil, which have had hydrogen shot into them to extend shelf life. (Thumbs-down to manufactured trans fats!)

Your Belly on (Saturated) Fat

The takeaway from the new microbiome research just confirms an older nutritional truism: all things in moderation. Yes, we can celebrate healthy fats like the omega-3s and monounsaturated fats—and I'll do just that in the next chapter. But in microbiome study after study, dietary fat, especially animal fat, was found to be the nutrient that most reliably promoted leaky gut syndrome. Here's what happens. The fat feeds some potentially unfriendly bacteria that live in the small intestine. These mostly "gram-negative" bacteria have an outer membrane that contains some very nasty molecules, or endotoxins (meaning toxins produced within the body itself). If these bacteria become numerous enough, in other words, well fed enough from bad fats and dense carbs, fragments of this membrane leak through the wall of the small intestine into the bloodstream and provoke an inflammatory response that can promote insulin resistance and weight gain.

Research has shown that people who consume a lot of saturated fat in their diet, as well as people who are obese, have gut microbiomes made up mostly of these gram-negative bacteria that produce these inflammatory endotoxins. In one study, the ingestion of 300 calories of cream, about six times the amount of cream in a cup of coffee, was able to cause the levels of these bacterial endotoxins in the blood to shoot up. This does not mean that some saturated fat in your diet is bad; in fact, some is necessary for cell membrane integrity. It's the excess that fuels a toxic gut.

Some researchers now suspect that diet may affect heart disease risk most tellingly by how it affects the composition of the microbes in our gut. This year, a group of Italian scientists suggested, "the way to a healthy heart may be through a healthy gut microbiota." As for the conventional argument that saturated fat causes heart disease by raising "bad" cholesterol levels in the blood, a lot of the older research has been reexamined, and there really is no consensus now about how much either saturated fat or LDL cholesterol contribute to heart disease. No matter what the final verdict is, your fat portfolio is in good shape with the Swift Diet, which is low in animal saturated fats and balanced in the healthy fats that I'll discuss more in the next chapter.

Mass-Produced Vegetable Oils

Just as human civilization learned to concentrate the calories of wild grasses in grain flour, it also figured out how to squeeze the fat in plants into oil form. We're probably aware of the olive oil we put on our salads, but we're often oblivious to the rivers of mass-produced vegetable oils, mostly soybean oil and corn oil, that run through our processed foods—in this country, totaling about twenty-eight billion pounds a year. For all the energy that the public health establishment has lavished on warning us about the dangers of saturated animal fats, it's likely the vegetable oils—especially soybean oil and corn oil—that are the bigger threat to health.

The problem is the disturbed balance between omega-6, which we consume in huge quantities in these oils, and omega-3, found most abundantly in cold-water fish, wild game and some nuts and seeds. Today, we eat far more omega-6 and far less omega-3 than our Paleo ancestors. As usual, when our diet strays too far from the way humans ate for millennia, the result is inflammation. Nature designed these two types of fats to keep each other in check. In excess, the omega-6 fatty acids get converted to pro-inflammatory hormones that can unsettle the gut and promote weight gain.

It gets worse. To keep the omega-6-heavy oils from going rancid over time, whether in the bottle or in processed foods like chips and commercial baked goods, the food industry pumps hydrogen into them, creating trans-fatty acids, or trans fats for short. They are bad news. They can "arm" the excess LDL cholesterol in your blood, making it more prone to turn into artery-clogging plaque. Unlike with saturated fat, our bodies haven't evolved to deal with trans fats—the process of partially hydrogenating these oils was introduced in the early 1900s. And the evidence suggests it can disturb a broad swath of human physiology. If we haven't pinned down the exact cause and effect, the consumption of trans fats tracks closely with increased disease. In the well-regarded Nurses' Health Study, a 2 percent increase in trans-fat consumption increased heart disease risk by a startling 93 percent.

The problems with soybean oil and corn oil begin long before the plants are processed in the food factory. The vast majority of these crops have been genetically modified (GM) to withstand what otherwise would be impossibly toxic amounts of pesticides. We're now routinely consuming plants containing certain proteins that the human system had never been exposed to before industrial agriculture got into the business of "improving" nature. Just how big a health hazard GM crops poses is a matter of intense scientific debate. For health and for weight and really for every reason I can think of, my prescription is to skip the processed foods and avoid GM food in general. Here is link to a non-GM shopping guide that is downloadable to your smartphone: http://www.nongmoshopping guide.com.

#4 Problematic Proteins

Digesting protein takes more metabolic energy than digesting fat or carbs, so diets higher in protein often do better in short-term head-to-head comparison of different weight-loss diets. Dr. Ludwig has found that the body's metabolism stays elevated on a higher-protein diet even after an individual meal has been digested, for reasons at this point we can only guess at. So I'm all for increasing people's protein intake *from plant sources*—legumes, for instance—if they can handle the digestive challenges. (We'll get to those in a moment.)

Historically, high-protein diets were thought to overburden the kidneys, but the current thinking is that this is only a serious problem if someone already has impaired kidney function. Protein from a serving or two a day of high-quality poultry or fish is fine. Fatty red meat, however, presents us with some health issues, and here the microbiome is deeply involved.

Meat: Metabolic Mayhem?

The research literature is stuffed with studies that analyze the dietary histories and medical records of large numbers of people and arrive at the unsettling conclusion that people who eat a lot of red meat are more likely to die before people who eat only a little. Keep in mind these studies are correlational—they establish that a behavior and a condition happen over the same period of time, but that doesn't mean one causes the other. And the meat they were looking at was the usual feedlot, industrially processed stuff. The results might have been different had it been higher-quality meat. Still, scientists have succeeded in identifying some potentially toxic ingredients in red meat that, taken together, explain why it may behave differently, and worse, in the body than poultry or fish and, specifically, why it may contribute to an increased risk for colon cancer. For one, the gut bacteria that feed on meat convert the nitrites in processed meats into potentially carcinogenic compounds. It turns out, they can create noxious N-nitroso compounds from non-processed meats as well.

Hot and Bothered

The invention of cooking meat, fish and poultry has on balance been a good thing for humankind, contributing to an increase in our brain size and saving us from countless pernicious bugs and parasites. But it too comes at a cost. When we cook animal flesh at very high temperatures, we're subjecting ourselves to some vile chemistry experiments. Especially when we grill or broil, we're creating a potentially carcinogenic family of compounds called heterocyclic amines (HCAs). We're also creating another class of molecules, AGEs or advanced glycation end products, formed when compounds in the meat bind with protein and fat. It's a natural process that occurs in us and in the animals we eat: when you leave a cut of meat out, it will "brown" over time, thanks to the accumulation of AGEs. The joint stiffness that we experience as we get older is another example. Our connective tissue is literally getting mucked up with AGE. And when we consume meat, especially meat cooked at higher temperatures, we increase AGE levels in our own body, increasing our susceptibility to heart disease, dementia and type 2 diabetes, in effect speeding up our own aging process! (Red meat has higher AGE levels than poultry, which has higher levels than fish—and bacon is the worst offender.)

The solution to the problems posed by both HCAs and AGEs is simple: Substitute fish for meat as often as you can and turn down the heat. Lower the temperature and increase the cooking time slightly when you grill, broil, roast, bake and stir-fry. Using a marinade when grilling can decrease HCA formation by up to 96 percent. And adding acidic ingredients like lemon or vinegar to your meat marinade will slow down the formation of AGEs. Cooking methods that make use of water, such as steaming and poaching, are safer yet. Culinary medicine to the rescue!

Microbial Mischief

In 2012 the gut bacteria made headlines when researchers at the Cleveland Clinic discovered a brand-new risk factor for heart disease. The bacteria ferment two nutrients, carnitine and choline, that are found in red meat and, in lesser quantities, in dairy and fish, and turn it into a toxic compound, TMAO (trimethylamine-N-oxide). High levels of TMAO in the body may "arm" the LDL cholesterol in the blood and make it more likely to do damage to the heart vessels.

Ammonia is one of the most common breakdown products of protein in the gut, and too much ammonia is suspected of damaging those all-important cells that line the wall of the colon. It may help account for the high rates of colon cancer in the West and the lower rates in parts of the world where people consume a greater range of plant fiber and less meat. In a real sense, the microbiome doesn't care what we eat. It will respond to whatever digestive challenge we send its way. But when we feed the wrong bugs with the wrong foods, we suffer the consequences. In fact, a brand-new study showed promising early results treating type 2 diabetes with a vegan diet, or what the Italian researchers described as a no-animal-protein macrobiotic diet. The researchers speculate that the improvements they saw are the result of the prebiotic fiber in the diet improving the balance of microbes in the gut.

Livestock Antibiotics

For some of us, the most harmful thing we ingest with our hamburger has nothing to do with the protein and everything to do with the way livestock are industrially processed. Eighty percent of the antibiotics in the United States are being fed and injected into animals, which may contribute—how much, no one knows—to a growing crisis of human antibiotic-resistant diseases. In the Unites States, according to the Centers for Disease Control and Prevention, some twenty-three thousand people die annually from illnesses related to antibiotic-resistant bacteria. The meat producers consider the routine use of antibiotics a cheap way to ensure that cattle, pigs and poultry don't get ill when they're jammed together in feedlots eating grain contaminated with their own feces. The industry term for this is CAFO (concentrated animal feeding operation). These regular low doses of antibiotics also promote weight gain in cattle, which should give you pause if you're reaching for an antibiotic at the first sign of the flu. There's even some interesting research suggesting that the stress hormones produced during these animals' short, unhappy lives can affect the humans who eat them. Remember, in some sense, we are what the animal ate and how it was raised!

Vote with Your Fork

Besides being a pressing public health issue, the way most animals are raised and slaughtered in this country is an ecological and moral disaster. The majority of crops in this country are grown to feed the animals we eat, most of it GM corn and soy. The methane produced by the livestock, and their collected waste, is a major contributor to climate change. Meanwhile the forests that act as "carbon sinks" to absorb greenhouse gases and counteract climate change are routinely cut down to make room for livestock pasture or for the farms to grow the food to feed the animals. You can educate yourself on these environmental and health issues on the Web sites for the Center for Food Safety (centerforfoodsafety.org) and Natural Resources Defense Council (nrdc.org).

It's not a pretty picture but you can improve it with your food-purchasing decisions, one meal at a time. To source humanely raised livestock, go to the Humane Farm Animal Care Web site, certifiedhumane .org, and look for the CERTIFIED HUMANE RAISED AND HANDLED label on the meats you buy. Alternately, check out Animal Welfare Approved and its Web site, animalwelfareapproved.org. The meats will be leaner and because the animals feed on grass, not grain, the omega-3 levels will be higher. It's my personal belief that you can and should eat a mostly plant-based diet, not only for your microbiome and your overall health but also for the health of the planet. At the heart of the concept of "nourish" is expanding outward your circle of concern, from "me" to "us." Another way of putting that: Vote with your fork.

#5 Gluten (and Other) Glitches

The word *gluten* comes from the Latin for "glue" and aptly, gluten does provide a familiar chewy texture to grain products. But while the pizza maker couldn't knead and stretch his dough into a pizza shape without it, it's hardly indispensable, which is fortunate because it may cause the body, and the belly, a lot of difficulty. According to the (conservative) statistics, 1 percent of Americans have the severe reaction to gluten, celiac disease, and 6 percent have non-celiac gluten sensitivity (NCGS), which suggests that gluten is a major problem. But my experience, shared by numerous colleagues, is that many of our clients feel and look better when gluten is excluded from the diet. With the explosion of gluten-free foods that have come on the marketplace in the past few years, and a growing familiarity with gluten-free whole grains like amaranth, buckwheat and quinoa as well as more familiar standbys like wild rice and (certified gluten-free) oats, excluding wheat, rye and barley is no longer *such* a big sacrifice to make.

Back in the Day

The gluten story begins, like a lot of dietary detective stories, with the introduction of agriculture about ten thousand years ago. When Paleo Woman began to eat ground-up wheat seeds, or flour, she was ingesting proteins stored in the plant for its own growth in addition to the starchy carbs that contain most of the calories. Because the human gut hadn't evolved to deal with gluten over the previous 99.9 percent of human prehistory, she couldn't completely digest it, and ten thousand years later, many of us don't do well with it either.

Over the past forty years, modern agriculture has selectively bred the traditional wheat plant to arrive at today's version, shorter, hardier and capable of producing higher yields. The gluten portion has increased either in size or in its capacity to react inside the body. Or both. These issues are still being debated. What is obvious is that our society is consuming more and more wheat, and grains in general, presenting challenges to digestion and overall health. Meanwhile, over this same period of time, the American gut was becoming less resilient because of poor diet, antibiotic use, and indeed for all the reasons I listed as root causes at the end of the first chapter. This mismatch has helped create the current epidemic of celiac disease and related disorders.

Gluten and the Microbiota

Scientists are still fleshing out the details, but it looks like the microbiota plays a crucial role in the gluten-wheat story. In our first years, the gut bacteria help educate our developing gut immune system to distinguish friend from foe. Being born by Caesarean section delivery or not being breast-fed or having a heavy exposure to antibiotics can all conspire to prevent the gut bacteria from becoming plentiful or diverse enough to "tune" the gut immune system so that it doesn't overreact to things like gluten. (Recall my gluten sensitivity story in the first chapter. I had the bad microbiome trifecta!)

We know there is a genetic component to celiac disease and the related conditions. But genes by themselves aren't enough. It's likely that a dysbiotic or out-of-balance microbiota can help turn on the "quiet" genes responsible for responding to gluten at any stage of life. A gut infection can disrupt the digestive ecology. Or, as we've already discussed, a processed-food-heavy diet fails to feed the bacteria that nourish the gut wall so that it becomes permeable or leaky, allowing microbes or food proteins into the bloodstream, where they can trigger an inflammatory immune system response.

Celiac Disease and "the Spectrum"

What we do know for sure is that the gluten-wheat epidemic is best seen as a spectrum of related conditions. They include celiac disease, non-celiac gluten sensitivity/intolerance (NCGS) and wheat allergies and sensitivities. Let's briefly examine them, one by one.

Celiac disease had been named and its symptoms studied going back to ancient times, but it wasn't until the middle of the past century that doctors figured out that gluten in the diet was in some people causing intestinal distress—constipation, diarrhea, bloating and abdominal pain—and damaging the gut's ability to absorb nutrients. It turned out that celiac was an autoimmune disorder, like rheumatoid arthritis or type 1 diabetes, in which the immune system, for reasons still not entirely understood, attacks the body itself. In the case of celiac disease, the immune system strongly responds to gluten and related proteins in wheat, rye and barley. It then mounts an immune response, making antibodies that attack not only the offending gluten proteins, but the gut's own digestive machinery, the microvilli in the small intestine.

Non-Celiac Gluten Sensitivity

But what about my client Susan and others like her? She didn't test positive for gluten antibodies and an endoscopy didn't reveal any damage to her microvilli. Was she, as her doctor surmised, simply mistaken that gluten was causing the problem, maybe even deluded? As medical science has only recently concluded, the answer is no. Over the past few years, academic leaders in gastroenterology, like Dr. Alessio Fasano at MassGeneral Hospital for Children and Dr. Umberto Volta at the University of Bologna, have published the research that has filled in our understanding of NCGS.

In the case of both celiac disease and NCGS, gluten enters the system and the gut gets dragged into a war. With celiac disease, the immune system feels so threatened, it calls out the heavy artillery, producing the antibodies that run amok and cause the autoimmune disorder. Not so with NCGS. Here, it's the immune cells housed within the gut that respond to gluten, and they in turn trigger the release of all-purpose immune cells called cytokines, which circulate in the bloodstream, causing inflammation wherever they go.

The gut is often affected—think of Susan's IBS-type symptoms—but sometimes digestion is untouched and the symptoms pop up only outside the gut; for instance, joint pain, skin eruptions like eczema, insulin resistance and the common hormonal disorder PCOS (polycystic ovary syndrome). As Dr. Fasano puts it, "The digestive system is not like Las Vegas. What happens in the gut doesn't stay in the gut." Considering that insulin resistance is one of the major drivers of weight gain (and PCOS, for that matter), not surprisingly, many of my gluten-sensitive clients come to me wanting to lose weight as well.

You'll remember in the preceding chapter how the brain and the gut are intimately linked, engaged in a never-ending two-way communication carried on by hormones and neurotransmitters. The NCGS-driven inflammation can distort that conversation and contribute to abnormalities in brain function that the mind experiences as anxiety or depression. There is some evidence that gluten intolerance may be linked to mental disorders like autism, ADHD, and schizophrenia. And some theorists, like the neurologist David Perlmutter, author of *Grain Brain*, believe that gluten-driven inflammation fuels age-related cognitive decline and even Alzheimer's. The evidence isn't conclusive; these stories are all unfolding.

However that plays out, we now appreciate that the more common gluten sensitivity can't be considered a form of "Celiac lite." People with celiac disease certainly may have more severe gut damage and consequently have problems absorbing the nutrients they need. But NCGS can also cause vitamins and minerals to be malabsorbed, which contributes to symptoms that can show up anywhere in or on the body. According to American celiac authority Dr. Tom O'Bryan, a major Swedish study looking at "gluten-related disorders" found that people with NCGS—inflammation only, no visible gut damage and no gluten antibodies—had a 72 percent greater than average chance of dying young, far worse odds than the people with celiac disease! The figures are alarming but the remedy is straightforward—eliminate the gluten.

Wheat Allergies and Sensitivities

But gluten isn't the whole story! Some researchers now suspect that a significant percentage of people who see their symptoms improve or disappear on a gluten-free diet are reacting not to gluten but to other components of the wheat plant. (Wheat has an estimated ninety-five thousand genes, about five times the number of human genes, so there are plenty of candidates.)

We know that at least a handful of these non-gluten proteins can trigger allergic responses in some people. An allergic response is different from a chronic autoimmune disease like celiac. As I'll describe in a little more detail later in the chapter, another set of immune cells goes into action, usually much faster, often causing symptoms within seconds or minutes of eating the problem food. Although these symptoms can be dangerous, even life threatening, they usually resolve relatively quickly with the careful elimination of the allergenic food.

A wheat sensitivity can be caused by the body reacting to some other component in the wheat; for instance, fast-fermenting carbohydrates called fructans. Here, the immune system isn't directly involved. IBS-type symptoms can result from eating foods like wheat that are difficult for a sensitive gut to digest. Again, more on these potentially problematic carbs—fibers like fructans and sugars like lactose—further down the MicroMenace list.

Many Problems, One Solution

As a clinician, I believe my practice is my living laboratory. I have witnessed dramatic improvement of symptoms, even their disappearance, when gluten and gluten-containing grains are eliminated from the diet. Sometimes this unfolds over a number of months; sometimes it's rapid—a matter of weeks, even days. The meal plans I'll provide in Chapter 7, "The 4-week Swift Plan," and the recipes in Chapter 8 should make this transformation as easy as possible.

But always, it comes down to the individual. For the person with celiac disease, the prescription is a meticulous, lifelong gluten-free diet. Someone with a milder sensitivity may want to experiment (that is, once she has completed the 4-week Swift Plan) to see how much gluten her system can tolerate. "Heritage grains," traditional grain strains with a more manageable gluten load, are becoming an increasingly popular option in the marketplace.

And finally, remember, not only are we limiting or eliminating problem foods in the Swift Diet, but, as we'll discuss in the next chapter, we're adding the healthy MicroMender foods that will make us and our guts more resilient and better able to deal with whatever potentially troublesome foods come down the digestive pike.

GLUTEN: COMING TO TERMS

Gluten-related disorders: an umbrella term that covers the spectrum of conditions and symptoms caused by gluten.

Celiac disease (CD) a.k.a. celiac sprue, nontropical sprue, and gluten-sensitive enteropathy: an abnormal immune reaction to gluten that damages the small intestine and interferes with nutrient absorption.

Non-celiac gluten sensitivity (NCGS): a term used to describe the presence of symptoms caused by gluten that don't meet the medical criteria for celiac disease. Symptoms may show up on the skin, in the nervous system, in the gut and on or in other organs.

Non-celiac wheat sensitivity (NCWS): a new diagnosis with symptoms similar to NCGS, but caused by a sensitivity not to gluten but to other proteins found in wheat.

Wheat allergy: the allergic reaction to those non-gluten proteins in wheat. The reaction is orchestrated by the immune system, which manufactures antibodies to attack these proteins.

GLUTEN GUIDANCE: SWIFT TAKEAWAYS

1. **Where to find it:** Gluten is found in the following grains and their grain products (flours, breads, cereals, crackers, pastas, etc.):

   Wheat: bulgur, couscous, dinkel, durum, einkorn, emmer, farina, farro, graham, kamut, seitan, semolina, spelt, sprouted wheat, wheat berries, wheat bran, wheat germ, wheat gluten, wheatgrass

   Rye

   Barley and barley malt

   Triticale (a crossbreed of wheat and rye)

2. **Be on the lookout:** Gluten can hide out in just about any processed food and in places you might least expect it; for example, malt, soy

sauce, natural and artificial flavorings. The list is endless! And if you're especially sensitive to gluten or have celiac disease, you also need to check your dietary supplements, medications, cosmetics and personal care products.

3. **Check your sources:** To help you figure out where the gluten is, check reliable resources such as celiac.com and celiaccentral.org or invest in the latest app for an up-to-date list of hidden sources of gluten.

4. **Explore wholesome gluten-free:** Here's a list of grains and pseudo-grains that are gluten-free—just remember, choose their whole food form (for instance, certified gluten-free steel-cut oats instead of instant oats).

> Amaranth
>
> Buckwheat (kasha)
>
> Corn (maize)
>
> Millet
>
> Montina (Indian rice grass)
>
> Oats (certified gluten-free)
>
> Quinoa
>
> Rice (all types)
>
> Sorghum
>
> Teff
>
> Wild rice

5. **Skip the glut of gluten-free junk.** The gluten-free marketplace has expanded exponentially, so we're now spending billions on gluten-free products that are nutritionally challenged. Be sure that your gluten-free products pass the same health litmus test that you'd apply to any food. Check out the product's nutrition facts and numbers to make sure it's not loaded with sugar, salt and nasty fats.

6. **It's about time!:** In a long-awaited step toward accurate gluten-free food labeling, the Food and Drug Administration (FDA) has released

its definition of *gluten-free* that food manufacturers must use. The rule defines *gluten-free* as having less than 20 parts per million of gluten, a small amount that won't trigger symptoms even in people with celiac disease. These new gluten-free labeling regulations are mandated as part of the Food Allergen Labeling and Consumer Protection Act of 2004, which requires food manufacturers to list the eight major food allergens. Wheat, one of the eight food allergens, is of course a major source of gluten: http://www.fda.gov/Food/ResourcesForYou/Consumers/ucm367654.htm.

#6 Lactose/Dairy: Sour Milk

The most common food intolerance in the world is to lactose, the sugar in all dairy products coming from cow, goat and sheep. For most people on the planet, including a majority of Asian Americans and African Americans, their bodies produce progressively less lactase, the enzyme needed to digest lactose, once they're weaned off breast milk. As they grow up, lactose-containing foods will contribute to those now familiar IBS-type symptoms—abdominal pain, excessive gas, constipation and diarrhea.

Undiagnosed sensitivities to lactose, fructose and gluten are the most common causes of the symptoms that send people to the gastroenterologist. In fact, some clinicians suspect that gluten intolerance often sets the stage for the usually less severe sensitivity to lactose and other food elements. It increases the chance that milk sugar compounds pass through the small intestine to the colon, where the bacteria there can ferment it into harmful by-products. These compounds and their by-products (or metabolites) can escape the gut into the bloodstream and cause systemic symptoms such as headaches and brain fog. (And some researchers think it's the opposite, that gut sensitivity to non-gluten compounds in milk, wheat and a number of fruits and vegetables gets mistaken for gluten intolerance.) For the lactose-intolerant consumer, reading labels on foods, dietary supplements and medications is a must to avoid the lactose in the dairy-based ingredients that could be lurking there!

I eliminate dairy completely in the first two weeks of the Swift Plan but allow for its reintroduction in the following weeks, including fermented milk foods such as yogurt and kefir that over time can increase the gut resiliency. I had to smile when I came across a new journal article from the Nestlé Research Center in Switzerland, which floated the theory that when the first herding tribes in the prehistoric Near East discovered how to ferment milk into cheese and yogurt, they were effectively seeding their guts with the lactic acid–producing bacteria, allowing them to digest the milk more easily.

#7 The FODMAP "Gang"

Now comes the tricky part. Certain high-fiber vegetables and fruits that help us build up gut health can, in some people, cause the very digestive symptoms they were designed to address. Remember the old Mae West line, "Too much of a good thing is wonderful"? Well, not true if your microbiome is in disrepair.

Around 2005, a pair of Australian nutritional scientists came up with an acronym that covered a collection of fibers and sugars that, inside the sensitive gut, can cause digestive distress by fermenting too rapidly and aggressively: FODMAP. (It stands for fermentable oligosaccharides, disaccharides, monosaccharides and polyols and yes, it would have been handier if they could have made it FOODMAP.) This bacterial over-fermentation creates an uncomfortable amount of gas and it may interfere with the colon's ability to maintain the body's "water table." It sends either too much water back into the system, creating uncomfortable bloat or, in more severe cases, diarrhea; or too little, causing constipation. So this idea of limiting high-FODMAP foods has become increasingly influential with nutritionists and some gastroenterologists, with good reason. In one major study, over 70 percent of the subjects lessened their IBS symptoms with a low-FODMAP diet. In early 2014, at the Gut Microbiota for Health World Summit in Florida, leading experts declared that the old view of IBS as a mostly psychological-driven disorder had to be replaced with a new understanding that emphasized the role of the gut bacteria.

EVERYTHING YOU ALWAYS WANTED TO KNOW ABOUT FODMAPS

FODMAP refers to carbohydrate-containing foods that are easily fermentable by gut bacteria. They can cause or contribute to gas and bloating in a sensitive gut. But many of them also provide important beneficial prebiotic fibers, so for most people, long-term exclusion from the diet is not advised. Note: "saccharides" equals sugar.

F = Fermentable

O = Oligosaccharides (fructans and galactans)

D = Disaccharides (lactose)

M = Monosaccharides (fructose and galactose)

A = And

P = Polyols (sugar alcohols): isomalt, maltitol, mannitol, sorbitol, xylitol

FINDING HIGH FODMAPS: THE SWIFT LIST

Sweeteners that are high in fructose: high-fructose corn syrup (HFCS), agave, honey

Sugar-free products containing polyols/sugar alcohols: gum, mints, candy, etc.

Gluten-containing grains and grain products: wheat, rye, barley

Fruit: apples, cherries, mangoes, nectarines, pears, peaches, plums, prunes, watermelon; dried fruits and fruit juices

Vegetables: artichokes, asparagus, beets, Brussels sprouts, cauliflower, celery, garlic, leeks, mushrooms, onions, scallions (white part only), snow peas, sugar snap peas

Legumes: peas, beans, and most soybean products except tofu

Nuts: cashews and pistachios

Dairy and dairy alternatives: lactose-containing milk and milk products, soft cheeses, soy milk and soy yogurt

Beverages: Chicory drinks (coffee substitutes made from chicory, high in inulin fiber), rum

Other: Inulin, chicory and other "FOS" (fructo-oligosaccharides) and "GOS" (galacto-oligosaccharides) ingredients added to foods and dietary supplements

Let's break it down. We've already covered two major FODMAP categories: lactose in dairy and fructose in high-fructose corn syrup and in fruits like apples, pears and watermelons, which have an especially high fructose content. Now we come to the fructans, related to fructose, which are found in gluten-containing grains like wheat, barley and rye. No problem there since we've already eliminated those grains from the Swift Plan.

But fructans (chains of fructose) also include the prebiotic fibers in vegetables that feed our microbial partners in the gut. Here's a partial list of these vegetables: artichokes, Brussels sprouts, garlic, onions and peas. The next category, the galactans, includes some more foods that feed our bacterial best friends: legumes such as lentils, black beans and soy. We'll cover some of these foods in the next chapter, "N: Nourish the Body, and the Belly." But in the Swift Plan, we'll go slowly to take into account the vulnerabilities of the sensitive gut. I'll gradually increase the amount of these healthy prebiotic foods over the course of Weeks 3 and 4, making use of the tastiest, healthiest ingredients in season.

Finally, the last FODMAP category is the polyols—sugar alcohols such as sorbitol and xylitol, which are found in sugar-free gums and candies.

Just like the sugar substitutes that we've already covered, eliminate them. But sugar alcohols are also naturally found in fruits such as nectarines and plums and vegetables such as cauliflower, snow peas and mushrooms. These whole-food polyols can be introduced into the Swift Plan over time.

FODMAP FUNDAMENTALS

1. Avoid the worst FODMAP villain: high-fructose corn syrup (HFCS)
2. Foods are ranked low, medium, and high in the FODMAP world depending on the amount of the fermentable carbs they include.
3. Each person responds to FODMAP foods in their own way. The same food that causes you gut distress may not bother your best friend at all.
4. The total FODMAP "load" is important. You may be OK with small amounts of certain high-FODMAP foods, but the cumulative amount could push you over the edge.
5. Eat fruit when it is just ripe, versus under-ripe or overripe.
6. The Swift Diet (Weeks 1 and 2) eliminates those FODMAPs that I have found most troublesome for my clients.

FODMAP research is ongoing, so it's best to check the FODMAP app— http://med.monash.edu.au/news/2012/fodmap-app.html—and my Web site, kathieswift.com, for ongoing FODMAP updates.

GAS: THE GOOD, BAD AND UGLY

Good Gas

Burping, belching, blowing or breaking wind/passing gas/flatulence (Latin: blow or break wind) are a part of *normal* digestion from eating a whole-foods, plant-based, fiberful diet. The average person in good health passes gas numerous times (about ten to twenty times) throughout the day.

Swift Solutions

Relax, we all do it! You might even see the humor in it, as some of us do, in a yoga or exercise class!

Bad Gas

There are a number of possible causes of *excessive* gas production, including:

- Eating or drinking too quickly. Instead, slow down your pace at the plate (you might even set a timer to monitor yourself for a while).
- Talking too much while you are eating. Try practicing reflective listening when dining and enjoy what others have to share.
- Eating when you're stressed out. Slow things down, pause, breathe, relax and, if necessary, distance yourself from the stressful situation.
- Food allergies and intolerances:
  - Wheat (gluten and fructans)
  - Dairy (lactose)
  - Gluten-containing grains
  - The FODMAP "gang"
  - Red meat and eggs (rich in sulfur compounds that may cause gas)
- Bubbly carbonated beverages. Switch to flat water.
- Chewing gum or sucking on candy. Avoid, as both sugar-free and sweetened types cause gas!
- Too much liquid with meals. Temper the amount of liquid you drink with a meal.
- Poorly fitting dentures. See your dentist!
- Weak abdominal muscles. Strengthen your abs/core with safe, simple exercises such as tightening your abdominal muscles by pulling in your stomach several times per day; consider wearing an abdominal support garment if exercise is too demanding.

Ugly Gas

Small intestinal bacterial overgrowth, chronic sinus problems and other medical conditions may be the cause of excessive bloating, belching, burping and gas. Be sure to check with your health care provider if gas, pain or bloating persists.

#8 Food Additives and Chemicals

About 70 percent of the food Americans eat can be considered highly processed. Food chemists have taken apart actual food, removed some ingredients and cooked up new ones in the lab to put back in their place. Consider the middle aisles of your supermarket or the drive-through window at your local fast-food joint as a giant science experiment. In former *New York Times* reporter Melanie Warner's *Pandora's Lunchbox*, she can't help being funny, in a gallows humor sort of way, as she describes the 105 ingredients that go into Subway's Sweet Onion Chicken Teriyaki sandwich, 55 of which, she writes, are "dry, dusty substances" that include things like disodium guanylate and calcium disodium EDTA. Subway's tagline? "Eat Fresh!"

Another mystery ingredient is azodicarbonamide, which Subway added to its bread to make it chewier, not surprising since it's commonly added to everything from shoe rubber to yoga mats to increase elasticity. In early 2014, Vani Hari, the Food Babe blogger (foodbabe.com), marshaled consumer pressure to persuade the company to remove it—it was already banned for human consumption in Europe and Australia because of a suspected link with respiratory problems like asthma.

Disturbing and ghastly as these food additives sound, I'm just as worried about some of the toxic chemicals that are sprayed on our produce or manufactured into our food containers and everyday household products. Triphenyltin (TPT) in pesticides and tribuyltin (TBT) in vinyl products have both been found to make lab rats fat. Bruce Blumberg, who researches these compounds at the University of California, Irvine, calls them "obesogens" and regards them as a hidden factor in the obesity epidemic. Other toxic compounds are even more widespread: bisphenol A (BPA) in plastic bottles and tin cans; perfluorooctanoic acid (PFOA) in Teflon and microwave popcorn bags; phthalates in shampoos. These are the "endocrine disruptors" that disrupt the sex hormones of lab animals. What they're doing to us is an open question. But public pressure forced the industry to remove BPA from baby bottles and Campbell's is removing it from their soup cans. Vote with your pocketbook, and with your blogs and tweets!

NOT-SO-SWIFT INGREDIENTS

Read food labels and avoid foods that contain the following additives and ingredients (and check out the Center for Science in the Public Interest's Chemical Cuisine Web site: http://www.cspinet.org/nah/05_08/chem_cuisine.pdf):

- Artificial colorings and flavorings
- Artificial sweeteners (acesulfame-K, aspartame, neotame, saccharin, sucralose, tagatose)
- Azodicarbonamide (ADA) (in yoga mats and hundreds of food products)
- Benzoic acid, benzoyl peroxide, and sodium benzoate
- Brominated vegetable oil (BVO)
- Butylated hydroxyanisole (BHA) and butylated hydroxytoluene (BHT)
- Caramel coloring that contains 4-methylimidazole (4-Mel)
- Carrageenan
- High-fructose corn syrup
- Hydrolyzed vegetable protein (HVP) and hydrolyzed plant protein (HPP)
- Monosodium glutamate (MSG)
- Nitrates and nitrites, including sodium nitrate, potassium nitrate, sodium nitrite and potassium nitrite
- Olestra
- Partially hydrogenated oils (trans fats)
- Polyols or sugar alcohols (erythritol, hydrogenated starch, hydrolysate, isomalt, lactitol, maltitol, mannitol, polydextrose, sorbitol and xylitol)
- Potassium bromate
- Propyl gallate

- rBGH and rBST—synthetic hormones in dairy products
- Sulfites, including potassium bisulfite, potassium metabisulfate, sodium bisulfite, sodium dithionite, sodium metabisulfite, sodium sulfite, sulfur dioxide, and sulfurous acid

#9 Alcohol: Salut, Sensibly

Drinking, especially heavy or binge drinking, can increase gut permeability and decrease its ability to keep what's supposed to be kept inside the digestive tract in. Alcohol consumption also ups the perils for women who are at high risk for breast cancer. And like most of the MicroMenaces, alcohol undermines both digestive health and weight loss. Many of the women I see for healthy weight management cannot afford the empty calories of one or two drinks a day. I think about my client Sharon, a classical musician in the Berkshires, who plateaued twenty pounds shy of the target weight she had set for herself. She was eating and exercising just as we had mapped out, but it was her routine of two glasses of wine at night to unwind, those extra 250 or 300 calories a day, that had impeded her progress. We agreed that she would limit the alcohol, no more than two drinks a week. It worked for her, as it has for a number of my clients, and that's the limit I've built into my Swift Plan in Chapter 7. You can space the drinks out or you could have both of them at a Saturday night dinner with friends.

ALCOHOL ALMANAC

One drink defined:

12 fluid ounces of regular beer (5% alcohol) *or*

5 fluid ounces of wine (12% alcohol) *or*

1½ fluid ounces of 80 proof (40% alcohol) distilled spirits

ALCOHOL HEALTH CONCERNS

Gut issues: too much alcohol can cause leaky gut, worsen reflux symptoms, affect bowel movements.

Breast cancer: many experts advise, no alcohol is best for a woman at high risk of breast cancer.

Weight: alcohol contributes calories, lessens inhibitions and may drive overeating.

Pregnancy: abstinence from all alcoholic beverages is advised.

#10 Suspect Foods

A recent report published in a prestigious journal notes that there has been a stealth-like rise in what are termed "adverse food reactions," in adults as well as children. These reactions include both food allergies and food intolerances. By now, you can appreciate that an impoverished microbiota is at least partly to blame.

Food allergies can quickly result in serious or even life-threatening situations. The immune system can go into overdrive responding to even tiny amounts of the problem food. Symptoms can occur within seconds to a few hours and affect multiple organ systems. If eating shellfish causes your lips or mouth to swell and you experience breathing problems or anaphylactic shock, you quickly learn to be vigilant about shellfish—and carry an EpiPen in case you are unknowingly exposed to the allergen. Some individuals are so highly allergic that even kissing someone who ate the food or being in the same room where the food is being prepared puts their life in jeopardy. For good reason, schools have strict rules about not serving peanuts to students.

THE ALLERGIC EIGHT: COMMON FOOD ALLERGENS

Eight foods that account for the vast majority of allergic reactions

- Eggs
- Fish
- Milk
- Peanuts
- Shellfish
- Soy
- Tree Nuts
- Wheat

But far more common than food allergies are the subtler food intolerances that are more difficult to pin down, often because the adverse reaction is delayed—for instance, it took me years to get to the bottom of my gluten issues. I admit that the terminology is confusing here. "Food intolerances" and "food sensitivities" are used more or less interchangeably, and experts in the field of allergy and immunology are still sorting out the precise definitions and nuances. But generally speaking, *food intolerance* is an umbrella term referring to adverse food reactions that have multiple causes, just as we talked about in the case of gluten and lactose intolerance. Food intolerances can be triggered by lots of things, including chronic stress, additives in the food supply such as sulfites or MSG and, of course, a dysbiotic gut flora!

BODY TALK

Here are some of the signs and symptoms that can be caused by adverse food reactions:

- Belly troubles: gas, pain, bloat, constipation, diarrhea
- Chronic congestion, coughing, runny nose, sneezing

- Fatigue and poor energy
- Hair thinning or loss
- Insomnia, sleep disruptions and trouble falling asleep
- Joint pain
- Mood problems, anxiety, depression, irritability, lack of concentration, brain fog
- Muscle aches and pains
- Skin changes: dark circles under eyes, rashes, eczema, rosacea
- Weight gain

Connecting the Dots

Some of my clients don't pay enough attention to making the connection between how they eat and how they feel. They risk going through life being made miserable by a food they could remove from their diets. Some of my clients pay *too much* attention and they suspiciously jettison good foods until they've whittled their diet down to a boring short list of "safe" foods. In both instances, the remedy is a healing-foods "elimination diet." The Swift Plan in Chapter 7 is an all-purpose elimination diet, but you can experiment on your own or with a nutritionist to work on specific dietary vulnerabilities. Remember, do not experiment with any food that you are seriously allergic to, unless you are working closely with an allergist.

Here are the rules to help you identify if a food intolerance is causing troubles. Use these guidelines when you *suspect* that a certain food or foods may be causing you to feel off.

- Choose one food to investigate at a time.
- Try the food on three separate occasions at least three days apart to account for any delayed symptoms.
- Take note of how you feel each time by keeping a detailed food and symptom journal. Maybe the food turns out to be innocent and the bad reaction you attributed to it was caused by something else, such as

a stressed-out stomach or sleep deprivation. Maybe the food *is* guilty. Eliminate it!

THE MICROMENACE HIT LIST

1. Dense carbs
2. Sugar and artificial sweeteners
3. Mass-produced vegetable oils
4. Problematic proteins (especially processed meats)
5. Wheat and other gluten-containing grains
6. Lactose
7. The FODMAP "gang"
8. Unsafe additives and chemicals
9. Alcohol
10. Suspect foods

Chapter 4

N: NOURISH THE BODY, AND THE BELLY

Lauren

A lot of my clients come to me as self-proclaimed sugar addicts. My client Lauren, an office manager for an insurance company in western Massachusetts, jokes that as a toddler her first words were "juice" and "cookie," not "Mama" and "Papa." She was able to keep her weight under control when she was younger, but over the course of her fifteen-year marriage, and meeting the demands of raising her daughter and holding down her job, she'd added sixty pounds to her "wedding weight." By the time she'd hit her forties, occasional digestive problems, especially persistent bloating and gas pain, had arrived and, along with it, eczema. Clearly, the candy and the baked goods weren't doing her any favors in the empty calorie department but, just as clearly, a disordered gut was compounding the problem. I put Lauren on the same 4-week Swift Plan that I'll describe in Chapter 7—lots of veggies, limited gluten-free grains and just enough fruit to satisfy that sweet tooth. She had been a late-night eater so I created a new family ritual for her. Every evening after dinner, Lauren, her husband and her six-year-old daughter would enjoy a piece of fruit. (I didn't care if it was pineapple, berries, citrus or whatever, as long as the peanut M&M's didn't come out.) Unlike every other attempt Lau-

ren had made to lose weight, this time her husband had agreed to go along for the ride, at least for the first four weeks. She felt like she had a partner. They've both been on it for a year now and Lauren has lost fifty pounds, ten pounds to go. Not surprisingly, her skin and abdominal issues have cleared up.

SELF-INQUIRY BOX

1. Has the budget "family" restaurant become the default family dinner? Has takeout taken over your weeknight dinner meals?
2. Are many of the vegetables in a well-stocked supermarket or farmer's market strangers to you?
3. Are there more packages in your pantry than fresh foods in the fridge?

L auren is like so many of the clients I've worked with over the years. She had some nagging digestive issues, IBS-type symptoms, and when we eliminated the gluten, they went away. But she's not Susan, whom we met in the previous chapter. Lauren's digestive issues were annoyances, not life changers. What they really were was a wake-up call. The way she was eating didn't suit the person she wanted to be or the life she wanted to live. Her diet was chockablock with MicroMenaces, especially the dense carbs that fed her lifelong sweet tooth. The result was the creeping weight gain that was draining her vitality. While it's likely she did have some degree of sensitivity to gluten, the bigger, underlying problem was that she was "allergic" to her processed-food and convenience-driven Standard American Diet. That's true for virtually all of my clients, women and men.

When I first met Lauren she asked me the question that as a nutritionist I've heard more than any other: *"Everybody tells me what I can't eat. But what can I eat?"* Now that we've covered the MicroMenaces in the previous chapter, we can answer Lauren's question. I call these "yes you can" foods the MicroMenders: working in concert with the microbiome, they help heal the gut and promote weight loss. Another common denominator: they are divinely delicious, as you'll discover in the recipes to come. Your gut bacteria may not care about this (although we are learning that there are taste buds in the gut!), but the pleasure you take in preparing and eating these foods is the best and most reliable incentive to stay on the healthy eating path.

Before we move on to the list, let me briefly explain the concept of "Nourish," the third step in the MENDS program. It means something bigger than "eat good food." That's key, of course, but as important as the "what" of eating is the "where." Lauren, like so many overscheduled women in this country, had fallen into the trap of relocating the family dinner to a nearby budget "family restaurant" or resorting to takeout menus. I see this at both ends of the age spectrum; for instance, the woman who's retired or whose kids have grown up saying to herself or her spouse, "Why bother; let's go out."

Practically speaking, this is usually a dietary dead end. Even if you're trying to order sensibly, the meals you get are likely to be full of cheap, mass-produced oils. Bread and bread products are going to be almost irresistibly arrayed around the table. Portion sizes will be fit for a lumberjack.

There's no avoiding it. The road to health and weight loss leads back to your own kitchen. Choosing the right ingredients and preparing them thoughtfully for *most* of your dinners is at the heart of what it means to nourish yourself and family, if you cook for more than one. Yes, it takes some time, which these days is a precious commodity. (In Chapter 7, "The 4-week Swift Plan," I'll take you through some smart, efficient shortcuts.) But study after study has demonstrated that home cooking pays dividends in health and weight loss. More than that, I would add, it can also be an antidote to the fractured ADD mind-set that our plugged-in, digitalized culture seems to encourage. When you cook, you have to pay attention to what you're doing, one thing at a time. (If not, watch out!) I like to say that cooking is a mindful act. In this book, you'll be introduced to a number of mind-body practices that can reduce stress and develop your powers of attention. Although we don't usually think about it this way, cooking is itself a powerful mind-body practice! (The workshop I launched five years ago at Kripalu, titled "Nutrition and Cooking Immersion," is now one of its most popular healthy-living programs. The students love the physical and sensory connection with the food.)

Here is the Swift Diet summed up in a picture—the Swift Plate. Half the plate is filled with non-starchy, often colorful vegetables such as carrots, spinach, kale, herbs and spices. A quarter of the plate is filled with starchy vegetables like sweet potatoes or acorn squash, complemented with whole grains such as quinoa or wild rice and fresh, seasonal fruit. And a quarter is lean, clean proteins such as wild fish and skinless turkey. You'll also see eggs and legumes as part of the protein picture. The droplet at the center of the plate completes the picture: healthy fats and oils, like extra-virgin olive oil, with a smattering of nuts and seeds.

Oftentimes, I advise clients to avoid processed foods. The advice is good, but it can be a little confusing since "processed" could mean anything

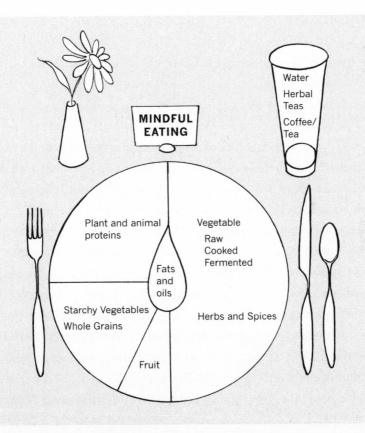

from extra-virgin olive oil to a bag of Doritos. Certainly, we do want to steer clear of food that comes packaged with a long list of hard-to-pronounce ingredients, some of which made an appearance in the previous chapter. As a general rule, we're shooting to eat food that has had as little "done" to it as possible. Another way to think about it is, your refrigerator and freezer should be full and your pantry nearly empty, save for spices and oils. The Swift Plate is what we're aiming for. In Chapter 7, I'll give you the step-by-step to get there.

The MicroMenders

As you'll see, whole plant foods are at the heart of my MicroMenders list, and the core of the Swift Diet. They're *that* valuable for three big reasons:

1. High in fiber
2. Low in calories
3. Rich in micronutrients and phytonutrients

Prebiotic and Probiotic Power

We've always known that foods rich in fiber are good for regularity, which is no small thing. But for a long time, the evidence was staring us in the face that fiber did more than that. Back in the late seventies, a famous British surgeon, Denis Burkitt, wrote a best seller in which he pointed out, much like the researcher Ian Spreadbury did recently, that traditional peoples who ate a plant-based diet high in fiber rarely developed our modern diseases of aging. (Burkitt proposed that the smaller the stool, the larger the hospitals!) In one 1959 study, for example, South African researchers looked through the records of over thirteen hundred autopsies of the Bantu people of South Africa and saw only a handful of instances of heart disease, our leading killer. Burkitt was convinced that fiber provided the single most significant heart-protective effect. But at about the same time he wrote his book, the American public health authorities were cranking up their campaign to warn us about the dangers of fat in the diet. Over the next thirty years, the story about what we should eat, fiber, was overshadowed by the one about what we shouldn't, fat.

The case against fat has gotten weaker, especially after a major meta-analysis published this year in the *Annals of Internal Medicine* couldn't find any connection between saturated fat consumption and heart disease. The case *for* fiber has only gotten stronger: improving insulin sensitivity and blood sugar, escorting excess cholesterol out of the system, cutting hunger. A 2013 analysis of twenty-two studies found a consistent association between fiber intake and fewer heart attacks and less heart disease. And yet, according to a recent University of Minnesota study, only 8 percent of adults and 3 percent of kids—you read that right, 3 percent—in this country meet the government's recommendation for consuming fiber in the diet. Those recommendations range from 19 to 38 grams a day depending on age and gender, but don't worry, when you follow Swift Diet meal plans and recipes, you'll get plenty. You don't need to count.

The new microbiome research has given us a clearer picture of how fiber operates inside the gut. The fibers that feed the friendly bacteria in the gut, for instance lactobacilli and bifidobacteria, are called "prebiotic." As we've discussed, these bacterial species maintain the integrity of the gut wall and tamp down inflammation. Jeff Leach, the cofounder of the American Gut Project, says we should take our cues from our Paleo hunter-gatherer ancestors and forage as widely as we can. Maybe it's our local farmer's market and not the savannah of Africa, but we can go farther afield and try out vegetables and fruits we're not familiar with, whose names we might not even know. Jeff calls it the "re-wilding" of the gut. The broader the range of fibers we consume, the broader the range of bacteria will be fed. In our inner ecology, just as in the ecology of the planet, diversity equals resilience. The more types of friendly gut bacteria we harbor, the better job of digestion the gut does, the less chance that a particular food or food component will cause localized gut upset or trigger a harmful inflammatory response.

Just about any vegetable or fruit you can think of can have a probiotic as well as prebiotic effect. That is, instead of being cooked or eaten fresh, they are prepared by putting them in a Crock-Pot or a mason jar and letting bacteria ferment them in there—before the bacteria inside your gut have a go at them! Certain common bacteria, like lactobacilli, break down the sugars in the plants into acids, preserving the food and imparting a distinctively salty, tangy flavor. When we eat them, fermented foods like sauerkraut and kimchi, both made from cabbage, provide fiber for our resident gut bacteria as well as a fresh shipment of transient bacteria just passing through. One fermented food, tempeh, made from fermented soybeans, delivers a fantastic fiber boost. Fermented milk products such as yogurt and kefir don't provide dietary fiber at all. But in every case, the new bacteria enhances the diversity of our gut microbes during their one-way transit and, in ways that scientists are just beginning to unravel, help the resident bugs do their job better.

PREBIOTIC POWER FOODS

A food that is prebiotic contains ingredients, mostly fiber, that the bacteria in the gut feed on, producing fermentation by-products that benefit our health. Here are some of the most potent prebiotic foods:

Almonds

Asparagus

Bananas

Burdock root

Cereal grains such as whole wheat, barley and rye (note: these grains contain gluten and can be a cause of food intolerance)

Chicory root

Endive

Garlic

Greens (especially dandelion greens!)

Jerusalem artichoke

Jicama

Kiwi

Leeks

Legumes

Mushrooms

Oats

Onions

Salsify

PROBIOTIC POWER BOOST

Here are some fermented foods to power up your digestive health:

Fermented vegetables (kimchi, sauerkraut, carrots, green beans, beets, lacto-fermented pickles, traditional cured Greek olives, etc.). You can ferment or culture any vegetable or fruit (lemon, lime and orange peel are delicious!).

Fermented soybeans (miso, natto, tempeh)

Cultured dairy products (buttermilk, yogurt, kefir, cheese) and cultured nondairy products (yogurts and kefirs made from organic soy, coconut, etc.). You may want to try making your own kefir. You can obtain the starter kefir grains from Cultures for Health (culturesforhealth.com).

Fermented grains and beans (lacto-fermented lentils, chickpea miso, etc.)

Fermented beverages (kefirs and kombuchas) and condiments (for example, raw apple cider vinegar)

Swift Shopping Tips: Here are a few of my favorite fermented food brands to get you started. Many excellent products are in the pipeline!

Trimona Yogurt, Real Pickles, Hawthorne Valley Farm sauerkraut and other vegetables, Divina Mediterranean (olives, etc.), South River Miso, Bragg Raw Apple Cider Vinegar, Redwood Hill Farm's traditional goat kefir, Lifeway's organic whole milk plain kefir.

Nutrient Density

As I described in the previous chapter, the calories of food are bound up in the macronutrients, the carbs, proteins and fats that fuel us and maintain the body's basic structure and metabolism. We couldn't live without them. But many of us eat more calories than our bodies need—we're overfed *and* undernourished. Really, healthy eating boils down to eating food with a generous amount of fiber and micronutrients such as vitamins and minerals, which play a macro role in making sure the body runs as cleanly and efficiently as possible. They protect us against metabolic wear and tear that over time can usher in the common diseases of aging—type 2 diabetes, heart disease, possibly cancer. As it turns out, many of the foods richest in micronutrients tend to be some of the lowest in calories. Vegetables in particular take up a lot of room on the Swift Plate, and in our stomachs, without contributing very many calories due to all that fiber and water. So when we combine the low calories with the big micronutrient payload, we get what's called "high nutrient density."

That's exactly what we want when we're trying to protect our health and, yes, lose weight. Compare veggies to a grain-based carb-rich food like a bagel or a bowl of pasta. Most of the calories in these foods are readily digestible starches. Carbs are the body's basic energy source, so a certain amount of carbohydrate is good and necessary, but, again, if we're taking in more than the body needs to function properly, we're converting these calories to fat—or, at any rate, stalling our weight-loss program—without any health gain in return. Whenever we can swap out foods that are less nutrient dense (like the grains) for foods that are more (you guessed it, vegetables), we're shifting our metabolism in the right direction. So, the formula for healthy eating and healthy weight loss is pretty simple: *consume as many micronutrients as you can and no more macronutrients than you need*. Too many empty calories means weight gain and inflammation. The road back to health, and healthy weight, is lined with nutrient-dense food, especially vegetables.

More on Micronutrients

Vitamins are organic compounds, part of the living world, made by plants or by animals who eat the plants (or by animals who eat animals who eat the plants). These vitamins are essential helpers for a range of physiological processes. Vitamin A, for instance, is involved in immune defense; B vitamins are the spark plugs in energy production. What they all have in common is that our bodies can't make enough of them—we depend on our diets to provide them for us. Minerals perform similar regulating functions in the body. They keep our bones strong (calcium, boron, vitamin K, etc.) and our cells able to maintain the proper fluid balance (potassium and magnesium). They're part of the inorganic, nonliving world, found in the soil and taken up by plants and the creatures who eat them (including us).

All of the nutritional elements we've talked about—fiber, vitamins, minerals, and the amino acids in protein—join forces to rid the body of metabolic waste and environmental pollutants. This multiphase physiological process is called "detoxification." Orchestrated by the liver in partnership with other organs like the skin, kidney, lungs and the microbiota, it's at work every second of our lives to maintain our resilience in the face of a toxin-tainted planet and food supply. This kind of nutrient-driven natural detox is especially important for people losing weight. As fat cells shrink, toxins that had previously been stored there escape into the system. Select nutrients (such as amino acids; vitamins C, E and the Bs; the minerals magnesium, selenium and zinc) neutralize these harmful compounds and speed their transit out of the body. Magnesium and potassium help to alkalinize the system when they're absorbed into the bloodstream and the tissues. The scientific evidence is mixed, but it may be the case that a diet rich in vegetables and fruits, healthy for so many reasons, may also help preserve bone health specifically, and tamp down inflammation generally, by assisting the body to maintain an optimal pH, or acid-alkaline, balance.

I confess, it bothers me when I see people selling the idea that you must buy their special "cleanse" or their boxes of detox powders, potions and pills. In my opinion, this amounts to boxing yourself into a pseudoscientific regimen that hasn't been well studied and might even get in the way of your body's own detoxification processes. The Swift Diet plan is the foundation for food-based detoxification!

Phytonutrients and Antioxidants

You may have come across the term *phytochemicals* or *phytonutrients*. These are organic compounds in plants ("phyto" means plants)—thousands of them as compared to the dozen or so recognized vitamins—which play an important role in protecting our health. We still don't know enough to say any of them are essential (as in, we would die without them) or to establish a recommended daily allowance the way we do with vitamins. But over the past few decades, scientists have been studying different tribes of phytochemicals, mostly the phenolics, especially the flavonoids and the carotenoids, to parse out their benefits. Phenolic compounds such as lutein in orange bell peppers, for instance, helps maintain eye health, and the lycopene in tomatoes appears to protect against cancer.

And finally, that brings us to *antioxidants*, a term that identifies compounds not according to their chemical family but by what they do for us. As the name suggests, they protect us from the ravages of oxygen. We need oxygen to live, of course, but in the course of the chemical reaction that converts oxygen to energy in our bodies, free radicals are created. These are destabilizing molecules that damage our DNA, which can lead to cancer and neurological decline, and they set in motion the accumulation of toxic metabolic waste products that often add up to chronic disease. Fortunately, we have our internal defense system, antioxidant enzymes that neutralize the free radicals.

We can also use some help, and this is where vegetables and fruits come into their own. They've evolved their own compounds to protect themselves against oxygen poisoning and the sun's ultraviolet rays. The same chemicals in plants and fruits that neutralize the free radicals also give them their distinctive colors, our tip-off as to which antioxidant phytochemicals they contain. They come color-coded and contain vitamins and minerals such as vitamins C and E, selenium and other antioxidant superstars! Luckily for us, humans have coevolved with plants, so when we eat them, these chemicals join forces with our own antioxidant defenses, sometimes directly, sometimes indirectly when the plant chemicals stimulate the production of our human enzymes.

Vegetables simply have no rival in the food world in terms of the number of species, the number of *families* of species, and the range of colors, textures and flavors. (For that matter, the genes in the plant world, like the genes in our gut bacteria, far outnumber those in the human genome.) This diversity puts them in a league of their own when it comes to enhancing health and weight management. The research is so strong and so consistent that a diet rich in vegetables and fruits pushes down the rates of chronic disease, the government's 2010 Dietary Guidelines for Americans recommends *at least* nine servings of vegetables and fruits a day. You can also use the Centers for Disease Control's fruit and vegetable calculator, which takes into consideration age, gender and physical activity: http://www.cdc.gov/nutrition/everyone/fruitsvegetables/howmany.html. Since vegetables are such low-calorie health-promoting powerhouses, the first two entries on my MicroMender list are devoted to them, non-starchy and starchy. I'll highlight a handful of both non-starchy and starchy vegetable groups in the pages that follow, but please don't get the idea these are the only ones worth eating. The full edible menu deserves its own veggie nutritionary!

#1 Non-Starchy Vegetables

Everything I've said about the virtues of vegetables in general goes double for non-starchy vegetables. They are the stars among the stars, with the highest amount of health-protecting micronutrients packed into the lowest number of calories. Besides the compounds that protect them from oxygen, they've got other valuable chemicals that ward off both dangerous soil microbes and animal predators. Some impart a sharp or bitter taste that animals generally don't like. But we've evolved side by side with the veggies in a clever way. Over the millennia these same sharp tastes, while they may take a little getting used to, are pleasing to us, and the compounds responsible for them bolster our own antioxidant defenses. And there's exciting research suggesting that one family of phytochemicals in particular, the polyphenols found in a wide range of vegetables, fruits and herbs (and tea, coffee and red wine) helps with weight loss. The polyphenols work to stabilize blood sugar and insulin levels, discouraging fat storage, and they're a favored food of a common species of gut bacteria associated with healthy body weight. By now, it might not surprise you to learn that a whole new research avenue has opened up that looks at the polyphenols not as antioxidants but as prebiotics that feed the good bacteria, which are in turn responsible for many of those vaunted health benefits.

POLYPHENOL PICKS

Here are few that make my list, and if you want to find out if your favorite foods are on the polyphenol hit parade, link to: www.phenol-explore .eu-reports.

Apples

Berries (all types) and dark fruit such as purple grapes

Citrus

Cocoa powder and dark chocolate (more than 70% cacao)

Flaxseed

Green tea

Herbs and spices: cloves, curry, ginger, peppermint, rosemary, sage, thyme, etc.

Olives, black and green

Onions

Pecans

Soybeans

And, as we've discovered, fiber is just as important an ally in health and weight loss. The fiber type that has been studied most intensively for its ability to feed our bacterial friends in the microbiome is called inulin, found in garlic, leeks, onions, asparagus, artichokes, bananas and chicory root. Consuming a range of plant fibers is our best bet, which is where the non-starchy vegetables, almost countless species in all shapes, sizes and colors, excel. They contain both soluble fiber—that is, the fiber that ferments in the gut—and insoluble fiber, which has a limited ability to interact with the microbiome and mostly passes through the system, enhancing regularity along the way. These terms are a little dated, even though nutritionists still use them. There are actually scores of different types of fiber that together combine to form a matrix that the body needs for optimal health and digestion.

There is a yin and yang to vegetables, as with almost everything else in the food world. The same fibers that enhance our digestive health, of which inulin is a prime example, can cause over-fermentation in the gut for people whose microbiota are seriously out of balance. As we mentioned in the previous chapter, that's why vegetables that are otherwise nutritional superstars find themselves on the FODMAP cautionary list on page 81.

Leafy Greens

Leafy green vegetables like kale, Swiss chard, mustard, collard, dandelion greens and spinach are packed with vitamin K, important for bone health and proper blood clotting, as well as magnesium and potassium, which relax the blood vessels and help maintain healthy blood pressure. These minerals are a counterweight to the salt (sodium) that's poured into our processed foods, which in some people can have the opposite effect, constricting blood vessels and raising blood pressure.

Purslane, a seasonal leafy green popular in China, Mexico and Greece, was found to have the highest levels of heart-healthy omega-3 fatty acids of any known edible plant, and ten to twenty times more melatonin, an antioxidant with possible anticancer properties, than in any other vegetable or

106 of 356 THE SWIFT DIET

fruit analyzed. For all that nutritional muscle, it has a mellow, lemony taste and mixes well in a salad.

Arugula is a leafy green that's actually a member of the brassica family but, unlike broccoli and cauliflower, it comes without any digestive baggage. And because it hasn't been cultivated on a mass scale until recently, it's still got most of the nutrient punch of the primeval plant. (As Jo Robinson explains in her excellent book, *Eating on the Wild Side*, most of the vegetables and fruit we eat today have been for centuries selectively bred for sweetness and increased calorie content.) Arugula's wild peppery taste tells you that some powerful compounds are at work here. The glucosinolates protect the plant against toxins in the soil and may protect us from cancer. This is in addition to the usual nutrient boosters you find in leafy greens: high levels of vitamin C, folate, calcium and iron. Add arugula and other wild greens to sandwiches, salads, to smoothies or as a colorful and edible garnish to your entrée and leverage the power of plants!

Two other families of vegetables belong among my non-starchy standouts. Yes, they can present digestive challenges for some, owing to their high FODMAP content, but when they're integrated into the diet, step by step, the payoff is truly "food as medicine."

Brassica Family

Vegetables in the brassica family, such as broccoli, cauliflower, Brussels sprouts and cabbage, serve up a full plate of vitamins, minerals and phytochemicals. (They're also called cruciferous, for their cross-shaped flowers.) They've probably attracted the most attention for a nitrogen-based family of compounds I mentioned a moment ago, glucosinolates, which may help prevent stomach, breast and prostate cancers. The brassicas are key players in an ensemble cast of foods and nutrients that help the body detoxify. A number of studies have found that broccoli consumption can reduce the levels of a harmful estrogen by-product that both raises the risk of breast cancer and, for some women, contributes to many of the unpleasant symptoms associated with perimenopause and menopause.

Allium Family

The members of the allium family—chives, garlic, onions, leeks, scallions—have a medicine chest's worth of medicinal properties between them, as well as a pungent flavor that makes them a culinary mainstay. In the phytochemical department, they're high in sulfur compounds, quercetin and anthocyanins, associated with anticancer, antimicrobial, antifungal and blood-thinning effects. Many of garlic's healthy compounds are bound up in a substance called allicin, which gives the plant its unmistakable aroma and is released when you let garlic stand for a few minutes after peeling. But as you learned in the previous chapter, garlic and onions are also members of the FODMAP family and are temporarily eliminated in Weeks 1 and 2; but no worries—other aromatic vegetables pinch-hit in the recipes.

White Vegetables: Overlooked and Misunderstood

Nutritionists have been so effective driving home the message that brightly or deeply colored vegetables are good for us—the carotenoids in carrots and red peppers, the anthocyanins in blueberries and beets—that sometimes white vegetables get overlooked in the mix. A mistake! Cauliflower, a mainstay of the brassica family, and mushrooms are a nutritional jackpot! Mushrooms, a tasty fungus, are one of the few great sources of vitamin D in the plant world. They're rich in minerals and they contain a number of cancer-fighting compounds that research science is just beginning to get a handle on. In Japan, more exotic and expensive varieties like shiitake and maitake have been prized for their health benefits for ages, but a few years back researchers discovered that the humble white button mushroom delivers as much or more antioxidant power. New research has also found that mushrooms exposed to sunlight can capture the ever-so-important vitamin D—we boost our intake of this vital nutrient when we consume them! Another fascinating fungus fact: the often-discarded mushroom stems make effective prebiotics, feeding our partner in gut health, the lactobacilli, in the colon. Whether it's a grilled portobello replacing a fat-laden burger and providing that umami taste and meaty texture, or crimini, white button, or shiitake added to stir-fries, soups, salads and pasta, those pale mushrooms can nutritionally light up a plate.

Non-Starchy Vegetables

Artichokes

Asparagus

Bamboo shoots

Beans (green)

Beets

Bok choy

Broccoli

Broccoli rabe

Brussels sprouts

Cabbage (red, green, Napa, savoy)

Carrots

Cauliflower

Celery

Chives

Cucumber

Eggplant

Endive

Fennel

Garlic

Greens (arugula, chard, chicory, collards, dandelion, endive, escarole, kale, mesclun, mustard, radicchio, romaine, spinach, tatsoi, watercress)

Jicama

Kohlrabi

Leeks

Mushrooms

Okra

Onions

Peppers (sweet bell, hot)

Purslane

Radish (daikon, red)

Rutabaga

Scallions, green tops

Snow peas

Sprouts (broccoli, sunflower, mung bean, etc.)

Squash (spaghetti, yellow-summer)

Tomatoes (cherry)

Turnips

Zucchini

Swift Tips

- These non-starchy veggies should make up the bulk of your plate—ultra-low calorie and super-high nutrient density! Feel free to include additional servings from this list in your Swift Plan if needed—for instance, an extra side dish of steamed greens or a crunchy raw salad. Let this be your first go-to list!
- Color-code your daily fruit and vegetable intake by including each of the following color groups: red/pink; yellow/orange; blue/purple; dark green; white/green; white/brown.
- Enjoy both raw and cooked vegetables as there are nutritional benefits to both—for example, glutathione, a powerful antioxidant, is far more plentiful in raw vegetables and fruits, while phytonutrients such as lycopene, found abundantly in tomatoes, become more available to the body when the food is cooked and topped with a touch of olive oil.
- Prioritize organic choices per the Environmental Working Group's "Dirty Dozen" list (ewg.org), see page 115.
- Be adventurous about new, interesting choices—orange cauliflower, rutabaga, tatsoi—and experiment with sea vegetables such as arame, hijiki and nori to boost minerals naturally.
- Choose fresh vegetables in season and shop at farmer's markets; support CSA (community supported agriculture) whenever possible.
- Don't love a particular vegetable? Try, try again . . . and after about the

fifth or sixth try, your taste buds will say yes—the same advice we would give to our kids!

#2 Starchy Vegetables

These are the root vegetables that store their nutrients underground in bulbous root structures—potatoes, sweet potatoes, beets—and they're joined by aboveground plants like winter squash, and corn and peas, which technically are fruits, not vegetables. What they all have in common is a lot of starch, the storage form of glucose in plants. And that's why, traditionally, starchy vegetables had a bad reputation. They pack more carb calories, gram for gram, at least three times as much as their non-starchy cousins. But what gets overlooked is that most starchy veggies are also loaded with vitamins, minerals and phytochemicals, so they still manage to be a fairly nutrient-dense package. When it comes to providing dietary ballast, sweet potatoes and peas, to mention two, are excellent replacements for pasta and bread.

Potatoes and Peas

The sweet potato, a tuber but not actually a member of the potato family, is every nutritionist's friend. The antioxidant beta-carotene, which gives it the nice orange color, may protect vision and boost immunity, and for pregnant women, the B vitamin folate is insurance against birth defects. But the humble russet potato, too often written off as the plant world's answer to junk food, is also a source of vitamins and minerals, and the skin bumps up the fiber. Add yellow and red potatoes to that mix and you have multicolored nutrition. The purple potato is a relative newcomer with an ancient pedigree. It's a great example of a "wild" food, a direct descendant of the original plant eaten by the Incas; compared to the russet, it's smaller and even more nutrient dense and delicious!

The problem with potatoes isn't the potato; it's what we do to them, turning them into processed foods like French fries or potato chips, or slathering them with sour cream and fake bacon bits. Potatoes are good examples of something called "resistant" starch, also found in unripe bananas and legumes. As long as the potato hasn't been overcooked to a starchy mush, when it cools, let's say in a potato salad, the structure of the starch changes, making it slower to digest. Instead of being quickly broken down and absorbed by the small intestine, it passes down to the colon, where it acts as a prebiotic, food for the friendly bacteria.

Peas are another quality starchy vegetable (if, technically, the seed of a legume) that doesn't get the respect it deserves, probably because some of us grew up eating the canned variety. They've got protein, vitamin K, crucial for bone health, and a first-rate package of vitamins, minerals and phytochemicals, including two, lutein and zeaxanthin, that protect against the sun's rays and age-related decline in vision. While more and more people are taking the time to shell fresh garden peas, snow peas and snap peas, frozen peas are a handy alternative that preserves most of the plant's nutritional punch.

Starchy Vegetables

Corn

Parsnips

Peas

Pumpkin

Plantain

Potato (purple, red, white, yellow)

Rutabaga

Salisfy

Squash (winter: acorn, butternut, hubbard, kabocha)

Sweet potato

Water chestnuts

Yam

Swift Tips

- Starchy vegetables contribute many valuable vitamins, minerals and substances essential for gut health and immunity.
- A tennis-ball-size serving partnered with some protein and lots of

non-starchy vegetables, along with some healthy fat, is the way to build your Swift Plate.

- Potatoes are on the EWG's Dirty Dozen list (see page 115).

#3 Fruits

Fruits, like vegetables, are nature's gift to humans, filled with micronutrients and fiber. Unlike vegetables, they haven't always been appreciated and sometimes they've even been maligned. The calories in fruit come mostly in the form of sugars, both glucose and fructose. We know that these sugars added to processed food are bad news, driving up insulin production, taxing the liver and promoting weight gain. But locked within the cellular walls of fruit, these same molecules break down slowly in the gut and, in modest amounts, are nature's answer to our sweet desires. One or two pieces a day should be fine in addition to the fruit you might add to a smoothie. As I mentioned earlier, even fruits with famously high sugar content, like pineapple, still have a relatively, and reassuringly, low carb density and glycemic load, thanks to all that fiber. Last year, in the pages of *The Journal of the American Medical Association*, Dr. David Ludwig surveyed the research literature and found that fruit consumption was associated with lower body weight and a decreased risk of type 2 diabetes. (I have always been pro-fruit, so I was glad to see the *New York Times* draw attention to Dr. Ludwig's study.) The exceptions are fruit juice and dried fruit, both with concentrated doses of sugar that can disturb a sensitive gut, drive up insulin and promote weight gain if consumed in excess. My recommendation: add a splash of an antioxidant-rich fruit juice (pomegranate, cranberry or wild blueberry) to seltzer, not more than a couple of ounces, or to a marinade, not more than a quarter of a cup. Limit the dried fruit to one small serving; for instance, a chewy fig or a coconut-rolled date instead of some processed snack food.

For people with sensitive bellies, those FODMAP compounds found in certain fruits can be a concern. That's why in Weeks 1 and 2 of the 4-week Swift Plan, I stick to lower-FODMAP fruits that are unlikely to cause belly upset—low-risk, high-fiber propositions. First, the berries—blueberries, strawberries, raspberries, cranberries. The phytochemicals in the flavonoid family that give them their deep and different colors are some of the most potent antioxidants yet discovered. Another group, the anthocyanins, are thought to have powerful anti-inflammatory effects. You've probably heard this story—blueberries in particular get a lot of attention. My friend John Bagnulo, PhD, MPH, much-loved nutritionist, farmer and environmentalist, conducted extensive research on blueberries and confirmed their "super food" status. And recent animal research from Texas A&M and the University of North Carolina is beginning to fill in the microbiome picture—in an animal study, the consumption of blueberries increased the number of friendly bacteria in the gut.

Another favorite is the kiwi, which deserves to be more popular. The green flesh of this fibrous egg-shaped fruit delivers a ton of tart flavor. Hidden inside is a huge dose of vitamin C and a range of other antioxidants. Included in the mix is a compound called actinidin, which, according to research published in 2013, looks like it may stimulate the growth of the gut's protective mucous lining. And who knew? Kiwi are grown not only in New Zealand (hence the name) but also in Maine!

Fruits

Apples

Apricots

Avocados

Bananas

Berries (blackberries, blueberries, cranberries, raspberries, strawberries, etc.)

Cherries

Clementines

Coconuts

Figs

Grapes

Grapefruit

Kiwi

Lemons

Limes

Mangoes

Melons (cantaloupe, honeydew, watermelon, etc.)

Nectarines

Oranges

Papayas

Passionfruit

Peaches

Pears

Pineapples

Plums

Pomegranates

Star fruit

Tangerines

Swift Tips

- Choose fruits in season for maximum taste, nutrition and thrift.
- Prioritize organic choices per the EWG's "Dirty Dozen" list (ewg.org).
- Bake fruit for a delightful dessert and top with spices such as cloves, allspice, nutmeg or cinnamon.
- Freeze fruit such as grapes or pineapple for a cool treat.
- Dried fruits (cranberries, dates, dried plums, figs, raisins) provide minerals such as calcium, iron, fiber and many phytonutrients. But go easy, as they're also a concentrated source of sugar and FODMAP.

The Lowdown on Pesticides: the "Dirty Dozen"

Frankly, we don't really know how much harm parts-per-billion pesticide residues are causing us. It's fair to say that corporate America isn't rushing out to do the studies that might prove that the combinations of chemicals that we consume with our produce are making some people sick or pose a real health risk to our children. But yes, ideally, you want to avoid fruits and vegetables that have been bathed in hard-core industrial pesticides. At a minimum, I'd avoid the Dirty Dozen, the nonprofit Environmental Working Group's famous roll call of the twelve most pesticide-laden foods in the supermarket (www.ewg.org/foodnews/summary.php), a list that has actually crept up to fourteen. Also worth checking out is their mirror-image list, the Clean Fifteen. Be aware, these lists are updated periodically, but if you download their app, you get the latest revisions.

Don't misunderstand. The Dirty Dozen are all great plant foods and frankly, I'd rather you have the "dirty" versions than none at all. But if you're able, get the nutrients without the industrial chemicals by buying produce labeled ORGANIC, and thanks to the mega food retailers who've embraced it, it's widely available. And, yes, expensive. But you can still significantly limit your exposure to the bad stuff; for example, by buying food that's grown locally and sold at the farmer's market. It's not worth fretting about achieving 100 percent food purity, and it's not possible anyway. (Remember that study I mentioned in the second chapter—"food fretting" was an eating style associated with overeating!) But by applying some pragmatic mindfulness when you buy your food, you can significantly reduce your toxic load.

Dirty Dozen Plus

Apples
Celery
Cherry tomatoes
Cucumbers
Grapes
Hot peppers
Kale/collard greens
Nectarines—imported
Peaches
Potatoes
Snap peas—imported

Spinach

Strawberries

Sweet bell peppers

Clean Fifteen

Asparagus

Avocados

Cabbage

Cantaloupe

Eggplant

Grapefruit

Kiwi

Mangoes

Mushrooms

Onions

Papayas

Pineapples

Sweet corn

Sweet peas

Sweet potatoes

POWER OF FOOD IMAGERY

Here's a digestive healing visualization exercise from Belleruth Naparstek (healthjourneys.com), who is *the* guru in the guided imagery field. Read the following script a few times, find a comfortable chair, close your eyes and imagine it! It will relax and reassure you about the healing power of food.

You're eating fresh vegetables and fruit. Imagine the carbohydrates breaking down to glucose that is delivered to your cells to burn as fuel. But the fiber in the food slows down the process, so it's clean and orderly and the sugar doesn't build up in the blood. Imagine the fiber massaging the gastrointestinal tract so it relaxes and gets rid of waste efficiently. Picture the healthy fats in the food building up the membranes that protect the cells and that allow messages to go in and out, directing essential jobs all throughout the body. As this food energizes you, makes you stronger, imagine the neurochemical communication between the digestive system and the brain, everything tuned to exactly the right frequency, like a two-way radio sending and receiving a perfectly clear signal. Let that series of images sink in. Allow the real purpose of what you eat to inform which foods you choose throughout the day.

#4 Legumes

Legumes like beans, lentils and chickpeas are the nutritional backbone of the world. The majority of humankind gets most of its protein from plants. Every culture has its own favorites and its own ways of preparing them. In the industrialized West, because we can afford it, we get most of our protein from animal foods, but we'd do well to go back to the plant, for ecological as well as nutritional reasons. Legumes are a relatively cheap, high-powered source, not only of protein but of fiber, minerals and vitamins. They are rich in folate, which reduces homocysteine, a measure of vessel inflammation and heart disease, and they contain a class of phytochemicals called lignans, which may lower rates of hormone-related cancers such as breast cancer and prostate cancer. And we've discovered that eating low-glycemic foods such as legumes at one meal keeps your insulin from spiking at the next meal, no matter what you consume. It turns out that the gut bacteria breaking down those plant fibers are largely responsible for this "second-meal effect." Although you may come across nutritional myths to the contrary, legumes are your friend when it comes to blood sugar.

For all that they do for us, keeping our weight down and protecting our health, legumes sometimes get a bad, and mostly undeserved, rap. Vegetarians were for years advised that they had to combine specific foods at meals, typically a legume matched with a grain, to get the necessary full complement of protein-building amino acids. The good news—you don't have to worry about particular food combinations at every meal. True, different plant foods have more or less of particular amino acids, but eating a wide range of protein-packing plant foods over the course of the day— legumes, nuts, seeds, gluten-free grains—will more than take care of your protein needs, whether you eat animal foods or not.

Soy can help out here as well. This legume has a full lineup of all of the important amino acids, a "complete food." But soy attracts its own bad press. Some people are allergic to soy and must avoid it at all costs. Soybeans contain isoflavone phytochemicals that mimic, mildly, the effect of estrogen, so the fear was that eating too much of it might stimulate the growth of hormone-sensitive cancers such as breast cancer. But the best current evidence says that, if anything, high-quality soy foods have a mildly protective effect. I am a fan of moderate consumption of organic whole-food soy, either fermented as tempeh or miso, or fresh in-the-pod edamame. But avoid the processed soybean oil and foods (textured soy protein, soy protein isolates and other junk soy) in those burgers, bars and chips that have infiltrated our food supply.

Here's another complaint about the legumes (and about the grains we cover in the next section). Advocates of meat-friendly Paleo diets like to point out that these plant foods contain "anti-nutrient" compounds, such as phytate, which interfere with the absorption of valuable minerals. In other words, these foods aren't as good as they look on paper and you'd better order that steak if you really want to satisfy the body's nutritional requirements. Well, phytate and its chemical cousins do reduce mineral absorption, so that part holds up. But the latest research tells us that phytate also serves as an antioxidant, cleaning up harmful oxygen free radicals generated by normal metabolism. So phytate and other anti-nutrients giveth and taketh away, yin and yang. And even cooler, friendly bacteria being fed by the fiber in the legumes help break down the phytate in the gut, freeing up some of those minerals to be absorbed by the system.

We've already discussed the major issue with legumes, those highly fermentable FODMAP compounds. They tend to be high in both fructans and galactans, which can irritate problem guts and, frankly, may contribute to a little unwanted gassiness in any of us. In the Swift Plan, we'll start out with easier-to-digest, lower-FODMAP legumes such as organic firm tofu and tempeh (a fermented food choice) and work up to the denser beans like black beans and chickpeas as the plan unfolds.

You can also avail yourself of some traditional methods of legume preparation that will begin to break down both the FODMAP compounds and the phytate. Less gas and more minerals—you can't beat that! So, for instance, soak the beans in a pot overnight (at least twelve hours), then rinse them off and cook them in fresh water. For the full treatment, place the soaked beans in a sprouting jar or sprouter and wait three to five days, until a small sprout appears, then cook.

If legumes sometimes require a little experimentation, they're worth it. They're valuable for what they have—nutrient-dense calories packed with fiber—and for what they don't have—the dense carbs or gluten that makes some grains so problematic. As the Harvard researchers discovered when they substituted one daily serving of beans for one serving of rice, switching from the grain to the bean is a major health upgrade, lowering by a third the risk of developing metabolic syndrome.

Legumes

Beans (adzuki, black, cannellini, chickpeas/garbanzo, Great Northern, kidney, pinto, etc.)
Lentils (black, French, green, red)
Peas (black-eyed, green, split, yellow)
Soy products (edamame [green soybeans], miso, natto, tempeh, tofu)

#5 Great Ancient Grains

You can have the best of both worlds, whole grains that don't contain gluten and are better tolerated by sensitive bellies. Best of all are the pseudo-grains, high-fiber, low-glycemic-load seeds that provide the feel and taste of grains without the gluten. Many of them have ancient and quite fascinating pedigrees: wild rice, amaranth, buckwheat and quinoa (pronounced "KEEN-wah").

A thousand years ago, Native Americans were harvesting wild rice, the seed of a tall aquatic plant, and the Chinese may have been eating it centuries ago as well. (So bound up was wild rice in the Native American culture that even today, in Minnesota, it can only be harvested from a canoe, according to state and tribal law.) The first European settlers in North America immediately took to its chewy texture and complex nutty taste. Today, it's often mixed with brown rice to increase the protein and B vitamins and up the flavor.

The consumption of amaranth may go back about eight thousand years. The tiny seeds of the plant were a nutritional staple of the Aztecs, who went so far as to mix them with blood in their religious ceremonies. The conquistador Cortés banned amaranth, as either food or religion, and cultivation of the plant went underground, only to reemerge centuries later in both Asia and the Americas. Today, the mild nutty-tasting seeds can be enjoyed in morning porridge, as a side dish or added to an entrée, or ground into flour or pasta. They're packed with fiber, protein, iron, zinc and magnesium.

Buckwheat's origins as a food go back to Asia, maybe five thousand years ago. It eventually made its way to Europe, and German and Dutch settlers brought it to the United States in the seventeenth century. Today, it's probably best known as the flour used to make the blini pancake. Roasted hulled buckwheat kernels are known as kasha. Combined with vegetables, they make a hearty and fiber-full all-plant meal. In any form, the seeds are a fine source of protein, iron, magnesium and B vitamins.

Over the past decade or so, quinoa has become the star of the ancient-grain world, available in supermarkets or upscale restaurants almost as readily as in health food stores. Breakout success has been a long time coming. It's been continuously cultivated for over five thousand years— the Incas ate it for sustenance, just as the Aztecs did amaranth. They knew what they were doing. Quinoa is a bona fide "super food," with all of the essential amino acids well represented, loaded with fiber and a great source of B vitamins and minerals such as magnesium and potassium. Maybe best of all, its crunchy texture and nutty flavor should put to rest any lingering longing for wheat. Not to mention, it is a super-swift-cooking grain!

Here's another good choice: oats, which I rarely recommended because so much of it was cross-contaminated with gluten. But because certified gluten-free oats are now available, that's much less of a concern. They're delicious, not only for you but for the friendly fellow travelers in your gut. Recent research shows that the beta-glucan compound in oats may be a potent prebiotic and that the polyphenols, also part of the package, have anti-inflammatory, anti-itching and possibly anticancer effects. With oats, as with any food, the less refined and the more packed with fiber, the better for you, so steel-cut oats trump instant oatmeal every time.

Gluten-Free Whole Grains

Amaranth
Buckwheat (kasha)
Corn (maize)
Millet
Montina (Indian rice grass)
Oats (certified gluten-free)
Quinoa
Rice (all types)
Sorghum
Teff
Wild rice

Swift Tips

- Soaking or sprouting grains may improve digestibility. Placing the grains in a fermented liquid (kefir, for example) can offer probiotic benefits.
- Add flavored tea bags, fresh/dried herbs, ground ginger, etc., to the cooking water for grains or use an organic vegetable broth.

- There are many delicious wheat pasta alternatives:
  - Noodles made from lentils, mung beans or black beans are loaded with protein and fiber.
  - Kelp noodles are another interesting alternative and very low in calories. They provide the mouth feel of a noodle and can be used in soups or salads.
  - Tofu shirataki noodles, made from konnyaku (yam cakes made from a Japanese plant's root) and tofu. Extremely low in calories, House Foods brand is verified GMO-free; prior to cooking, pour boiling water over noodles to enhance freshness.
  - Veggie "pasta"—spaghetti squash or other noodles you can easily make on your own from carrots, zucchini, yellow squash, etc., with a fun and inexpensive spiral noodle gadget!

#6 Animal Protein: Lean, Clean and Not-So-Mean

By now, you've gotten the idea that I'm passionate about plant food, for nutritional and ecological reasons. But sustainably and humanely produced animal foods merit a place in the Swift Diet. To borrow a term I love from the nutritionist blogger Ashley Koff, I'm a "qualitarian." While I have a deep respect for the vegetarian option, I endorse fish and modest amounts of skinless poultry and lean red meat, in smaller quantities, let's say 4 ounces or less as a typical serving.

Let's start with eggs, the marquee item in this category. For years, eggs were demonized in the public health war against dietary fat. Egg yolks do in fact have a lot of cholesterol in them, but now we appreciate that dietary cholesterol doesn't seem to pose a significant heart-health risk. The humble egg contains plenty of protein and the yolk is a nutritional mother lode—vitamin A, riboflavin, choline, carotenoids, which together protect and nourish brain and eye health.

NOT EGGXACTLY!

There are a lot of confusing terms on egg cartons these days, so here are my rules for egg selection:

1. If you can get fresh eggs from your own chicken or the farm down the street where the chickens get to roam freely and eat bugs, dirt and anything else they find, go for it!

2. If you purchase eggs at the supermarket, look for organic, certified humane eggs. The ORGANIC ensures that antibiotics were not used (hormones in poultry are forbidden by law). The labels CERTIFIED HUMANE or ANIMAL WELFARE APPROVED mean the chickens were allowed to roam around and were not caged in crowded conditions. Terms such as *cage-free*, *free-roaming*, *pasture-raised* and the like are loosely defined and unregulated.

Fish Tale

Fish, as we've discussed, is the best source of the omega-3 fatty acids EPA and DHA. Without some fish in the diet, or supplements that contain fish oil or algae, it's tough to get enough of these fatty acids in the diet from whole foods. Our bodies don't do a great job converting the ALA in seeds and nuts into DHA and EPA. And there's a mountain of research literature parsing out omega-3's specific health benefits, including studies showing that societies that eat a large amount of fish, the Japanese and the Scandinavians, for example, or a moderate amount, as in the Mediterranean regions, on average live longer and healthier lives than the rest of us.

For all of its health advantages, and sheer deliciousness, fish can be a fraught subject. Mercury toxicity is a real concern, especially as you move up the food chain to the predator fish like swordfish and mackerel. I like how my friend Dr. Cynthia Geyer, the medical director at Canyon Ranch in the Berkshires, puts it: "Throw the big ones back." The small, oily fish like anchovies, sardines and herring are great, safe bets, as are shellfish like oysters and mussels. Beyond that, choosing between popular larger species like salmon, cod and bass is tough. If it's a wild fish, is it being overfished and the stocks depleted? If it's a farmed fish, has it been raised in unsanitary conditions, leached of its natural nutrients, and treated with antibiotics? The calculus changes from species to species and sometimes from month to month. The best advice I can give is to check the Web sites and apps of either the Marine Stewardship Council (msc.org), Monterey Bay Aquarium's Seafood Watch (seafoodwatch.org) or the Natural Resources Defense Council (nrdc.org) for the best and latest information on supporting sustainable fishing.

Where's the Beef?

There's no question that poultry and red meat are excellent nutritional packages: rich sources of protein, minerals and B vitamins. In the case of red meat, we want the leanest cuts available, such as filet mignon or sirloin. Bison is leaner still and growing in popularity, and game meats in general are a good way to go. With poultry, I suggest losing the skin, tasty as it is. The concern about the saturated fat in the skin has waned in the past few years, but fatty tissues in the animals we eat are a repository of toxins, hormones and antibiotics, so I still proceed with caution. Pork, if the meat comes from humanely raised pigs, is acceptable. For all the meats we're discussing, I'm concerned about the industrial processing of animals and the nutritionally inferior and potentially harmful product that this system produces. To search out the more humane alternatives and improve the nutrient quality of your food (grass-fed beef has some omega-3 fatty acids, almost absent in the grain-fed animal), visit the Humane Farm Animal Care's Web site, certifiedhumane.org; or Animal Welfare Approved's Web site, animalwelfareapproved.org.

Animal Protein

Dairy (cow, goat, sheep): cheese, kefir, milk and yogurt
Eggs
Fish, shellfish

Poultry (chicken, duck, turkey)

Red meat, lean cuts (beef, lamb, pork)

Wild game (buffalo, ostrich, venison, etc.)

Swift Tips

- Whenever possible, purchase organic, certified humane animal foods.
- Avoid high-mercury fish such as shark, tilefish, swordfish, and king mackerel.
- Dairy products that contain lactose (milk, yogurt, soft cheeses, etc.) may bother the sensitive gut. Greek yogurt and hard cheeses are lower in lactose and can be included in moderate amounts for the person who is dairy tolerant.
- The type of animal may matter when it comes to allergy potential. For example, you may tolerate goat and sheep products but not cow's milk products. Even the breed of cow may make a difference, as proteins from the milk of the Jersey cow may be less allergenic than from the more common Holstein cow.
- Use safe cooking methods with fish, poultry and meat, such as low-temperature (less than 350°F) baking, roasting, poaching, and stewing. If you grill, use a marinade and do not char the flesh food, to avoid creating toxic compounds.

Dairy is excluded from the Swift Plan in Weeks 1 and 2. There are non-dairy alternatives available in the marketplace, but be sure to check on the ingredient list, because some of these food items may contain sugars, gums, gluten and other ingredients that irritate a sensitive belly and you are better off without them.

Nondairy Alternatives

Beverages (organic, unsweetened/plain: almond, coconut, hemp, rice, soy, etc.)

Cheese (made from almond, rice, soy, etc.)

Yogurt (organic, unsweetened/plain: almond, coconut, hemp, rice, soy)

Swift Tips

- Experiment with making your own nondairy products if the choices available in your supermarket contain problematic ingredients.
- Explore my friend Caroline Nation's Web site, myfoodmyhealth.com, and whole-foods chef Leslie Cerier's book, *Gluten-free Recipes for the Conscious Cook*, which is chock-full of interesting recipes, like how to make your own nondairy milks and other delicious vegan staples.

#7 Healthy Fats

While the scientific battle rages over animal saturated fats, we can soak up the benefits of whole-food fats that can and should be part of a gut-friendly weight-loss program . . . in moderation. All sources of fats and oils that exist in nature are a mix of fatty acids, some of which the body can make and others that are essential, meaning they must come from the diet.

As we discussed in the previous chapter, the omega-3s are the stars of the polyunsaturated fats, the PUFAs. They've been the most intensively studied for their health effects and found to benefit everything from helping to stabilize heart rhythm to reducing platelet "stickiness" in the blood, to lifting mood and supporting brain health.

The monounsaturated fats (MUFAs), in nuts, seeds, olives, olive oil and avocados provide antioxidants that may help protect cells and other compounds in the body, such as cholesterol, from excessive oxygen damage. Remember, we can use all the help we can get from plants to protect ourselves from the side effects of oxygen.

Cutting-edge research points to saturated fatty acids as one of the most potent disruptors of the gut micro-ecology, so I'm cautious about them. But it's a case-by-case proposition. In the Swift Plan, I restrict the amount of meat in the diet for a number of reasons that we discussed in the previous chapter, not just because of saturated fat. Dairy is its own story. In the plan, I'll introduce it gradually, as an option, over the course of Weeks 3 and 4. The fermented dairy products, primarily yogurt and kefir, can be great belly allies. And I'm OK with small amounts of whole milk or half-and-half in the coffee—that's how I take my one cup in the morning. Again, I'm more concerned with quality. Ideally, you should go with organic milk from pastured cows, and my preference is whole milk or cream that contains the valuable fatty acid CLA (conjugated linoleic acid), which may help improve insulin function and aid with weight control. Keep in mind that skim and low-fat milk have correspondingly higher levels of milk sugar, lactose, which, as we discovered in the previous chapter, comes with its own problems.

The saturated fat in tropical oils such as coconut oil and palm oil and cacao butter is another special case. These oils contain some medium-chain saturated fatty acids, which behave differently in the body than the marbled fat on a sirloin steak. Coconut products have become quite trendy. Sometimes these "flavor of the month" foods don't fare so well over time. But based on everything we know now, they're delicious choices to include in reasonable amounts.

Seeds

In the plant world, walnuts have a good supply of ALA/omega-3s, but otherwise, it's the small, edible seeds where you find it: chia seeds, ground flaxseeds, hemp seeds and pumpkin seeds. That makes sense. Seeds are a plant's storehouse of nutrients, ready to supply a new plant that takes root. They're even more nutrient dense than nuts (most of which are technically seeds, of the larger variety), rich in the good stuff: protein, minerals and essential fats. Seeds are enjoying a well-deserved boom right now, especially chia seeds. Aztec warriors used to eat them to keep up their energy on long marches. Today, we're more likely to add seeds to our smoothies to fill us up without adding too many calories.

Nuts

Nuts are more than the sum of their MUFAs and PUFAs. (I hope you enjoyed saying that sentence to yourself.) Nuts like almonds, pecans and walnuts are packed with minerals and the antioxidant vitamin E. The skin of these nuts is rich in flavonoid phytochemicals that support the immune system. The whole package tests out as a major health boon. In the famous Nurses' Health Study, which tracked over one hundred thousand women for decades, replacing carbs in the diet with the same amount of calories from nuts lowered the risk of heart disease by about a third. And numerous studies have found that eating nuts regularly is a reliable predictor of a long life span! When it comes to gut health, the fiber in nuts is a major plus, both the type that enhances regularity and the type that prebiotically feeds our friends in the gut microbiota.

With all that going for nuts, you might think you could eat as much as you like without regard to calories. Over the years, that's certainly what a lot of my clients thought. When we would put our heads together to figure out why they weren't making the weight-loss progress we had expected, the problem often turned out to be the nuts. Dietary fat, any kind of fat, contains over twice as many calories per gram as carbs or protein. There is *some* truth to "calories in/calories out," even if it's far from the whole story. (I've always been suspicious of a handful of small studies that suggest you can shrink the size of your belly by sipping tablespoons of vegetable oil every day.) So, sorry, no blank checks. You'll get a reliable read on how much is not *too* much of a good thing in the recipes in the last chapter. Let's take a look at a couple of my favorite healthy fat sources that are noteworthy when it comes to gut health and healthy weight.

Almonds

Almonds are mentioned quite a few times in the history books, and even in the Old Testament. That's fitting because almonds are particularly distinguished nuts. They've got the usual fine lineup of nut nutrients—magnesium, vitamin E, a collection of anti-inflammatory and possibly cancer-fighting flavonoid phytochemicals. And they've got more than the usual amount of fiber, 3 grams per ounce, which makes them excellent prebiotic candidates. A study in 2014 found that eating about 2 ounces of almonds a day for six weeks significantly increased the populations of our two most reliable friends in the microbiome, the bifidobacteria and lactobacilli.

Avocados

A luscious fruit that because of its low sugar and creamy texture is usually considered a vegetable, avocados are a rich source of monounsaturated fat, vitamin E and potassium, more than you'll find in a banana. They do contain a fair number of calories, about 300 for a nubbly Hass avocado, but I'm not so concerned about people inadvertently eating too much. They're not nearly so portable as nuts! And although you might not associate the rich-tasting, creamy avocado with fiber, it's loaded, about 13 grams, mostly the soluble kind that forms a gel in the gut. In a 2013 study out of Loma Linda University, adding half an avocado to the lunches of the overweight volunteer subjects significantly increased their feelings of fullness, or satiety, after the meal, suggesting they would be less prone to between-meals snacking.

Fats and Oils

Plant:

Avocado
Coconut, unsweetened (coconut manna, flakes, shredded)
Nuts, raw or roasted, unsalted (almonds, Brazil, cashews, macadamia, peanuts, walnuts, etc.)
Nut butters, raw unsalted
Oils (cold expeller-pressed: extra-virgin olive, grapeseed, virgin coconut, walnut, etc.)
Olives (black, green)
Seeds, raw (chia, flax, hemp, pumpkin, sunflower, etc.)
Seed butters, raw unsalted (pumpkin, sunflower, tahini, etc.)

Animal:

Butter
Cream
Ghee (clarified butter)

The Swift Diet on Fat

1. Eat whole "fat" foods: avocado, coconut, olives, nuts, seeds, nut and seed butters.
2. Choose cold expeller-pressed oils and use the one that best fits your cooking needs. Store oils in a cool, dark place.
3. Moderate your saturated fats and choose the highest-quality meat and dairy products (butter, cheese, ghee, kefir, yogurt, etc.). The way livestock is raised affects its nutrition and overall healthiness!
4. Avoid mass-produced vegetable oils and trans fats—soy, corn, cottonseed, partially hydrogenated oils and products containing these ingredients.
5. Avoid high-temperature cooking especially with certain fats and oils; for instance, extra-virgin olive oil. Refer to the kitchen cooking guide found at Spectrum Organics' Web site if you do turn up the heat: http://www.spectrumorganics.com/?id=116.

#8 Herbs and Spices

Pound for pound, or I should say ounce for ounce, nothing beats the antioxidant power of herbs, the strong-flavored plants we use to season our foods, either in whole-leaf form, such as basil or mint, or ground up as spices. Usually, a food's antioxidant activity is measured in the test tube, which leads to different results depending on which measuring technique is used, and raises the question of how much of this ability to mop up free radicals actually translates to metabolism inside the body. A 2012 study out of the University of Florida helped answer that question. The study subjects ate a number of spices—the amount that you'd get in a spiced dish, not a concentrated supplement—and then they had their blood drawn and tested. If they had eaten turmeric, rosemary, cloves or ginger, their blood produced significantly fewer inflammatory cells after being exposed to oxidized cholesterol, compared with the subjects who hadn't consumed those spices.

I know this sounds technical, but imagine, and please only imagine, that you'd eaten a plate of fried chicken. The spices that proved to be the most potent in the Florida study would limit the inflammatory fallout in your bloodstream. And we know, inflammation, besides promoting disease, also drives weight gain. The polyphenol phytochemicals in these spices help keep insulin in check and feed the good gut bacteria.

But maybe the best weight-loss assist that herbs and spices offer us is their pungent flavor. Humans have a hunger for taste. When we honor our "taste hunger" by cooking with nutrient-dense herbs and spices instead of eating sugar-and-fat-and-salt-laced processed foods, we pamper our palates to guide us to healthy weight. In fact, some research suggests that the flavors in herbs and spices modulate gut hormones that regulate hunger so that when we eat a flavorful meal, we reach fullness faster, with fewer calories. Some hot spices (and spicy vegetables in the pepper family) may even temporarily turn up the metabolic furnace a degree or two so that we burn calories more efficiently! Here's a look at a couple of my favorite herbs and spices.

Turmeric

Turmeric is a plant in the ginger family. When its underground stem is cooked and ground up, turmeric gives both curry powder and some mustards their yellow color. Its warm yet slightly bitter taste is one of the foundational flavors of the cuisines of South Asia, where the plant's medicinal properties have been appreciated for centuries. Modern research looking at the chief polyphenol in turmeric, curcumin, has found evidence for broad anti-inflammation effects. It's a valuable nutritional ally in the fight against metabolic syndrome, a constellation of common chronic problems like insulin resistance, high blood pressure and weight gain around the middle, all driven by inflammation. And add a bit of black pepper, as this helps boost absorption of curcumin!

Mint and Aloe Vera

The fragrant, refreshing taste of mint is welcome in a salad, in tea, iced or hot, or as a perky ingredient in homemade pesto. Loaded with minerals and phytochemicals and easily grown in an herb garden, fresh mint has been used for relief of digestive symptoms for centuries. It can quiet IBS-type symptoms and it can also be useful as a diuretic, to flush out toxins. Modern research is looking at both mint and aloe vera as antifungal agents. One 2013 study found that an extract from the fresh leaves of the aloe vera plant seemed to inhibit the growth of *Candida albicans*, a common and troublesome fungus that often resists conventional drug therapies.

#9 Drink Up!

Our bodies are mostly water, about 70 percent, so hydration is, of course, essential. Unless you're lost in the desert, it's not likely that you'd let yourself become so dehydrated that your life is endangered, but if you're not paying attention, it's easy not to drink enough to keep your gut happy and functioning properly. Water keeps wastes running through the system the way they should, especially important on a high-fiber diet, which, without adequate irrigation, can actually block things up. Constipation is an invitation to all sorts of digestive maladies and, as I'm sure we all know, it feels miserable. Here's a basic hydration guideline: drink whenever you feel thirsty. Thirst is a good indicator of your fluid needs. Many factors affect hydration requirements, such as age, exercise, environmental conditions and medications. A general guide to calculate your approximate daily fluid needs: divide your body weight by two. That gives you a rough estimate of the total number of fluid ounces you need daily, and good news, all fluids count in hydrating the body! There are also physical signs that give clues about your fluid needs; for example, your urine should be a light, straw color (note that B vitamins, beets and some medications may discolor urine). Clean, filtered water should be your beverage of choice, but let's take a look at some other beverages that you can enjoy, with a few caveats.

Coffee and caffeinated black tea are often viewed with suspicion in holistic health circles. Typically, they're among the first items on the "thou shall not" list that comes with the latest "cleanse." Well, I'm a pragmatist.

Yes, too much caffeine can pump up the stress hormones and upset the gut. But there's no convincing evidence that a limited amount—for instance, the option of one daily cup of coffee or a few cups of tea on the Swift Plan— causes any harm. But pay attention. If you notice that even one cup is bothering your digestion, do without!

Over the past few years, the research on coffee and tea has actually shifted to studying the positive effects, mostly attributed to the polyphenols. Coffee has shown preliminary promise in reducing the risk of both Parkinson's disease and type 2 diabetes, and evidence for other benefits is brewing. White, green and black tea all contain caffeine, but black tea has the stronger dose—the leaves are fermented, which liberates the caffeine. A particular polyphenol compound, EGCG (epigallocatechin gallate), found most abundantly in green tea, has been shown, mostly in animal and cell culture studies, to increase the sensitivity of insulin response and to help keep blood sugar levels stable. That should help with weight loss, in theory anyway, which is why you'll find it in lots of weight-loss supplements. Generally speaking, I'm not a fan of these supplements. You never know exactly what you're getting, and some of the ingredients could be harmful. But I'm all for tea, black, green or white—a few cups a day is fine.

Herbal teas are a wonderful treat with medicinal benefits, and no caffeine. Cinnamon and chai tea (without added sweetener) deliver sweetness and can improve blood sugar; hibiscus tea is good for the vascular system. Growing in popularity, red or rooibos tea contains compounds that have been found to lower stress hormone levels. Ginger and peppermint tea, along with teas that contain a mix of herbs, have gut-soothing effects and can be used for occasional help with constipation.

As we discussed in Chapter 3, when it comes to alcoholic beverages, it's best to limit yourself to no more than two drinks a week. Try a splash of bitters, good for digestion, in seltzer with lemon or lime in place of an alcoholic beverage.

MORE WATER PLEASE!

- Treat yourself to a new water filter to minimize heavy metals and industrial chemicals. Check out the Environmental Working Group's Web guide to water safety and water filters (www.ewg.org/research/ewgs-guide-safe-drinking-water).
- Invest in a portable glass water container or water infuser bottle to take with you when you are on the go.
- Avoid purchasing water in plastic containers for your health and the health of the planet.
- Add fresh cucumbers, ginger slices, citrus wedges or fresh-fruit ice cubes to add a flavorful zing to your water.
- Bubbly waters can cause more gas for some people but can also be soothing to other digestive tracts. Keep in mind that club soda has added salt while seltzer is sodium-free.

#10 Sweet, Not Sorry: Chocolate and Honey

Chocolate is made from the cacao bean, which has a sky-high concentration of a particular group within the polyphenol family, the flavonoids. It sounds too good to be true, but in study after study, the consumption of dark chocolate has been found to reduce heart-disease risk factors, lowering blood pressure and improving insulin sensitivity. This isn't a case of having your chocolate cake and eating it too. Avoid the sugary, fatty desserts and stick to pure dark chocolate—I recommend at least 70 percent cocoa/cacao solids. The higher the percentage of cacao, the lower the sugar. A couple of small squares a day shouldn't add up to enough calories to interfere with your weight-loss progress. If you can't limit yourself to that, skip the chocolate altogether.

Honey is more than a natural sweetener. It's an all-purpose food that is also a medicine. For over twenty-seven hundred years, it's been used as a topical treatment for burns and boils. An antimicrobial when it's applied to the outside of the body, when it's consumed it becomes an inflammation fighter on the inside. It helps to lower the levels of prostaglandins, chemicals made throughout the body that can cause blood vessels to constrict and blood platelets to clot too strongly. Honey does contain fructose, so it's capable of disturbing some FODMAP-sensitive guts. Use it sparingly and source a raw, local honey. But unlike table sugar, it actually serves as a prebiotic—food for the friendly bacteria.

Before we leave the topic of sweet nourishment, let me mention a few other sweet ingredients besides honey that you'll find in my pint-size pantry: blackstrap molasses (a nutrient dynamo that our grandmothers blessed), 100 percent pure maple syrup and coconut sugar. If a recipe calls for a touch of sweet, I'll use these instead of the white stuff!

#11 Fermented Foods: Cooking with "Cold Fire"

I've saved fermented foods for last, to set them apart a bit. Here we're not talking about a specific type of food but rather a particular way of preparing it, what Michael Pollan calls cooking with "cold fire." Using a few simple kitchen implements, such as a Crock-Pot and some mason jars, we're creating an environment where bacteria, and sometimes fungi, can begin the process of breaking down more complex nutrients into simpler ones. Basically, we're "predigesting" the food, re-creating in the kitchen what goes on in the gut every moment of our lives!

In the case of fermented vegetables, it's bacteria that's already on the plant that goes to work on the sugars and starches, converting them into compounds such as lactic acid, acetic acid and carbon dioxide. Whatever or however we're fermenting—vegetables (sauerkraut, beet kraut) or fruit (pick your favorites) or soy (miso, tempeh, tofu) or milk (yogurt, kefir)—the process preserves the food from spoiling while giving it a distinctively tangy taste. Conjure up the salty crunch of sauerkraut or the refreshing pucker of unsweetened yogurt. But for most of human history, fermenting food was more a matter of survival. It's how food could be stored over the winter (or in the case of milk, in summer) before refrigeration or canning. And yet over time these bacterial cultures became an important part of human culture. Traditional societies still invest a lot of their identity in these foods—kimchi in Korea or yogurt in the Georgian foothills of Eurasia. And today, these same foods are enjoying a renaissance with people who never grew up with them. They've acquired artisanal chic! This is how author and teacher Sandor Katz, the Johnny Appleseed of the "fermento" movement, describes the allure in his book *The Art of Fermentation*: "Between fresh and rotten, there is a creative space in which some of the most compelling flavors arise."

Actually, a lot of the food and beverages that we routinely enjoy are fermented at some stage in their production: coffee, black tea, chocolate, cheese, bread, wine, beer, ketchup, soy sauce. But for the MicroMenders list, I'm interested in foods where the bacteria are still hard at work when we consume them. The fermentation process boosts their nutritional value, breaking down "anti-nutrients" that can interfere with mineral absorption and often increasing the levels of B vitamins. The live cultures themselves interact with our own gut bacteria in interesting and not entirely understood ways. Even though the food bacteria mostly passes through and out the digestive system in a matter of a few days or weeks, the home-team microbiome still seems to benefit from the visit.

In one intriguing experiment, a leading researcher, Washington University's Dr. Jeffrey Gordon, found that the resident bacteria in mice were able to ferment a wider variety of dietary fibers after they had been exposed to a strain of bacteria commonly found in yogurt. Something is going on with the microbiota to explain the studies that have found, for instance, yogurt consumption associated with a lower risk of developing type 2 diabetes or that adding kimchi to the diet can reduce cholesterol and blood sugar levels. In animal studies, fermented foods have shown promise as an immune system booster as well, even inhibiting cancer cell production.

In my clinical experience, fermented foods can be a valuable ally in helping my clients overcome gut issues such as IBS symptoms and GERD, and even lose weight. It's difficult to tease out the effect of these foods by themselves. But, as I mentioned in Chapter 2, new research showing that the consumption of yogurt can change brain function or that kimchi can protect memory in mice is telling us that we've just begun to scratch the surface of what these foods can do for us.

Here's a brief sketch of some of my favorites.

Sauerkraut

Sauerkraut is certainly the best-known fermented vegetable dish. Back in the eighteenth century, Captain Cook forced his men to eat it on those long South Sea voyages so they wouldn't come down with scurvy—the fermentation preserves the vitamin C. And one of sauerkraut's active compounds, sulforaphane, looks to have cancer-fighting properties. And maybe most important, it just tastes good! Use a mason jar for a small batch or a Crock-Pot for a larger one and follow the almost foolproof directions laid out by Sandor Katz: "Chop, salt, pack, wait." (See my Pink Sauerkraut recipe on page 248.) Remember, you don't have to restrict yourself to the traditional combo of cabbage leaves plus juniper berries and caraway seeds. You can ferment most any veggie this way. I recently went to a fermentation workshop offered by a progressive-minded hospital, Fletcher Allen in Burlington, Vermont, and we fermented green beans, garlic, radishes, carrots, lemons and limes and had a blast in the kitchen! Not only is it good for your gut, but it's good for the environment (less food waste) and good for your pocketbook (you can buy produce on the sale rack!).

If you are going the store-bought route, your best bet is the refrigerated section of a health food store (those live cultures need to be kept cool). Read the label: it should say FERMENTED. If it says PASTEURIZED, that's a deal breaker: the cultures have been wiped out by pasteurization. RAW, CULTURED, NATURALLY FERMENTED—these are words to look for and the ingredient list should be simple. For example, Real Pickles brand of naturally fermented and raw organic ginger carrots contain: carrot, ginger, filtered water, unrefined sea salt—and that's it!

Tempeh

Making it yourself requires a starter mold and a MacGyver touch with the oven, so I confess I leave the DIY to Katz and buy the refrigerated little rectangular cakes at the local health food store. And this Indonesian whole-soybean food is very healthy indeed, with more protein, fiber and vitamins than its soy cousin, tofu, with a chewy texture and an earthy, slightly sweet taste. You can add it to almost any dish or use it as a meat substitute. In general, fermentation agrees with soy. It eliminates the gassiness that so often accompanies eating legumes of any type. And research done in Java, where tempeh first made its appearance in the 1700s, suggests that tempeh can build up the gut's resistance to infection, lowering levels of diarrhea caused by food poisoning.

Kefir

Kefir comes from the Turkish word *keif*, which translates as "good feeling." That should give you an idea how highly this slightly sour fermented milk drink is valued in its homeland in the Caucasus Mountains. The drink is a storm of probiotic activity thanks to the "grains"—actually a matrix of proteins, lipids and sugars—that drive the fermentation process. Because the proteins in kefir have already been partially digested, it's often a good choice for the lactose-intolerant. For anyone, it's an excellent source of B vitamins, as well as calcium, phosphorous and vitamin K—a milk cocktail for bone health! A number of studies have found antifungal and antibacterial properties in kefir, and one study showed that bacterial strains from the beverage have potential as a treatment for an inflammatory colon condition, colitis.

Swift Summary

So now you should have a pretty good picture of the foods that are and aren't part of the Swift Diet. If we eliminate or markedly cut back on the MicroMenaces discussed in the previous chapter and we pump up the

MicroMenders in this chapter, we've got a lifelong food template that could be summed up this with these 5 Fs:

Fiber: This is the quintessential food element to nourish your microbiota. Focusing on diverse sources—have another look at the Swift Plate—is the way to go!

Free: Food that is free of toxic ingredients and won't cause adverse reactions.

Flexitarian: Plant-centric but including some sustainable fish and high-quality lean meats and poultry for a diversity of flavors and nutrients.

Foraged: Scout some "wild foods" and "weeds" that are close to the ancestral vine to populate your plate.

Fermented: Reinoculate your gut with fermented foods that help the resident gut microbiota do its job.

Full-Circle Nourishment

In this chapter, we've talked about how to choose your food wisely with your weight-loss goals and your health in mind. But as we discussed at the end of Chapter 1, these decisions can have an enormous ripple effect. They connect you to the farmers who grow the food and the soil in which they grow it. When you take the trouble to buy produce that is organically or locally grown (and your local farmer may likely be producing fresher and more environmentally friendly food than what is labeled ORGANIC in the supermarket), you're not just buying good food; you're buying good soil! As my colleague Dr. Daphne Miller has described in her brilliant book, *Farmacology: What Innovative Family Farming Can Teach Us About Health and Healing*, soil that hasn't been blasted with chemical pesticides and chemical fertilizers contains a richer community of soil microorganisms—bacteria, fungi, nematodes—which in turn is more likely to produce nutrient-dense food. (Researchers from Washington State University were able to establish this using state-of-the-art DNA sequencing technology!)

Let's step back and appreciate this daisy chain. Your food choices support farming practices, which support a soil microbial community. That community in turn builds more nutritious plants, which feed a community of bacteria in your gut, which supports your own health and weight loss. The ecology of the soil is intimately connected to the ecology of your digestive system. Talk about full-circle nourishment!

Chapter 5
D: DIETARY SUPPLEMENTS

Nancy

Nancy, thirty-five, works as a high school counselor in the Berkshires. She has two boys under the age of ten. With all that going on, she rarely has time for exercise and she put on about fifty pounds over the past fifteen years. She also has disturbing digestive symptoms, which is why her local physician directed her to me. It didn't take too long to discover that Nancy's diet, otherwise fairly healthy, was loaded with gluten. With my guidance, she immediately eliminated that and she discovered a new world of gluten-free foods such as black-bean pasta and coconut wraps. After the first three months, she was beginning to slowly drop weight and her IBS symptoms abated somewhat. But her gut was still seriously off. She would go to work every day wondering if she could make it to a bathroom in time if the urge to go came out of the blue. I recommended Nancy take some sophisticated urine and stool tests to see if we could uncover any nasty microbes that might be responsible for her problem, but nothing showed up. It goes that way sometimes. I put her on a multi-strain probiotic and a broad-spectrum digestive enzyme supplement to ensure that the nutrients she consumed were being properly absorbed. It's helped even if I can't say why—neither her physician nor I can pinpoint exactly what's wrong with her gut. But Nancy has gotten enough relief from her symptoms that she can invest her newfound energy in exercise, and she continues to reap the benefits of the dietary changes she has made. To date, she's dropped twenty of the fifty pounds she intends to lose. She's convinced that the probiotic has helped her drop the weight. I told her that the latest research on probiotics and weight loss suggests she may be right.

SELF-INQUIRY BOX

1. Do you have a collection of supplements in your kitchen cupboard even though you have little or no idea what you're supposed to take them for?

2. Are you (rightly) suspicious of the "magic bullet" weight-loss ads you see on TV? Do you wonder if there are reputable supplements out there that might actually help with weight loss?

3. Are you aware that supplements can interact harmfully with some prescription medications, even with some other supplements?

L iving in a clean environment *and* eating fiber-rich plant foods to support the microbiota *and* adopting a sustaining lifestyle (we'll discuss that in the next chapter), there'd hardly be a need to supplement anything! But, as you may have noticed, our world, and often our lifestyles, fall somewhat short of perfection. And so I've found, particularly with clients who have health vulnerabilities, a prudent use of supplements can be a strategic way to shore up a weight-loss or digestive healing program that may have sprung a few leaks. Nancy's story is a great example.

But let me say up front: there is no one miracle digestive or weight-loss supplement that comes close to the power of "food as medicine." I am a supplement minimalist! But, you may ask, what's wrong with loading up on everything and anything that might possibly help you reach your goals? Here's the answer. At least once a week, a client will come into my office and unload a shopping bag of supplements on my desk—all products that they have heard about from a well-intentioned friend, from a health food store employee, or from surfing the Web. These pills and powders are supposedly going to boost their metabolism, lift their brain fog, spark their lagging energy and fix their bloated belly. And yet when we carefully go over their food and supplement diaries, I often find that many of these supplements aren't doing anything beneficial and may even be making their symptoms worse, not to mention depleting their finances! Willy-nilly, taking a smorgasbord nutrients and expecting the complex machinery of human metabolism to run better is naive.

Supplement Support

Now let's talk about the right way to use supplements. It's *not* about taking a random walk down the aisles at GNC or Vitamin Shoppe. Supplementation often requires the skill of a credentialed nutritionist or physician trained in integrative medicine, especially important if you've been diagnosed with a medical condition or are taking any medications. Together, you and your health care provider will come up with a strategy that considers only the supplements backed up by the strongest supporting research and that takes into account your personal medical history, family history, genetics, diet, medications and even lab findings. In this context, supplements can be a powerful tool to help soothe digestion, cool the fires of inflammation and stoke your energy.

Two of the most common questions that my clients ask:

How do I know if I need a supplement?
How can I tell if a supplement is working?

The body will sometimes provide physical clues in the form of various signs and symptoms that reflect unmet nutritional needs. For instance, a deficiency in B vitamins can lead to a wide range of symptoms in the mouth—a sore or inflamed tongue, gingivitis, or cracks in the corner of the mouth. Over time, it can lead to neurological problems or show up in sub-tler signs having to do with energy or hair or nails. There is no substitute for being mindful here and monitoring any significant changes in how you feel.

Frankly, it is often difficult, sometimes impossible, to know if a supple-ment is helping you. But by keeping track of when you take a supplement and how you feel, you may be able to find a pattern of benefit. Let's say you marked down on your calendar that you started taking 250 mg of magne-sium on September 20, when you were regularly having problems sleeping. On November 20, you write that insomnia is now only an occasional issue. On the flip side, this kind of log-keeping should be able to uncover if the supplement is causing side effects. Hopefully, they are mild and tolerable. If not, drop the supplement—theoretical benefit is never worth real-world harm. Here, digestive upset is probably the most common side effect. And sometimes herbal supplements can have a paradoxical effect as well. You take something to help you sleep and it keeps you up instead. Every person is biochemically different!

Laboratory tests have their place in the self-care universe. I'm talking about sophisticated tests that your physician may not give you when you come in for a checkup unless you specifically ask for them. In combination with the standard lab tests that measure kidney and liver function, they'll give you and your health care provider a fuller picture of what's going on in your body. They may well uncover evidence of a nutritional deficiency that can be addressed with the right supplement or of a health vulnerability that responds to the right combination of diet and supplements.

When it comes to weight and well-being, one test in particular leaps to my mind, the TSH, or thyroid stimulating hormone, test, which mea-sures thyroid function (see the Swift Basic Prevention Tests on p. 145). The thyroid gland is a kind of thermostat that regulates the metabolic rate of the entire body. When it slows down, from Hashimoto's, a common autoimmune disease, or perhaps from assault by environmental toxins over time, the consequences can be a laundry list of symptoms, including, most prominently, weight gain and fatigue. Addressing low-thyroid with diet, supplements and, if necessary, medications is a book in itself, but the first place to start is with a TSH test, or better yet, a full thyroid panel. I get one every year.

But diagnostic testing doesn't begin and end with thyroid. Let's say you have a high level of C-reactive protein, a marker for systemic inflammation and a risk factor for heart attack. You would be wise to try botanicals like turmeric and ginger, and omega-3 fatty acid supplements, all of which have anti-inflammatory effects. High levels of homocysteine, a protein that is a marker for heart disease, can indicate that the body isn't properly making use of the B vitamins it takes in. Taking supplemental B vitamins in the right form makes sense. For example, methylated forms of B_{12} (methylcobalamin) and folic acid (L-5-methyltetrahydrofolate) are more accessible to the body than some of the common forms tossed in multivitamins and B-complex vitamins.

I am often asked by clients, "What tests do you recommend my doctor order for me?" Here's a list that I developed with my friend Dr. Cynthia Geyer, the medical director of Canyon Ranch in the Berkshires, that lays out the lab tests that we consider important baseline measurements for health and wellness. However, keep in mind that no one test is a tarot card for health or illness. We're looking to find the patterns that emerge from analyzing all your laboratory data—it is critical for clinical decision making! Besides the tests, I've included a few thoughts on supplements to consider, in addition to dietary and lifestyle upgrades.

Swift Basic Prevention Tests

High-sensitivity C-reactive Protein (HsCRP) Test

What it measures:

• Marker of general inflammation in the body.

*Optimal Level:**

• Less than 1.0

What it tells you:

• HsCRP can be elevated for various reasons, including early response to infection, excess body fat, or other conditions. If elevated, it should be rechecked to confirm. Consider anti-inflammatory herbs and omega-3 supplements.

Hemoglobin A1c (glycated hemoglobin) Test

What it measures:

• Also referred to as A1c, this is an average blood glucose over a three-month period.

*Optimal level:**

• 4.8–5.4 percent

What it tells you:

• Blood sugar regulation is essential to health, so get A1c checked in addition to your fasting blood glucose (optimal level: 65–85 mg/dL).
• If elevated, consider soluble fiber supplements such as acacia or gluco-mannan (konjac root).

Fasting Insulin Test

What it measures:

• Insulin is a hormone produced by the pancreas that regulates blood sugar. It escorts glucose from the blood into the cells, where it can be used for energy.

---

* These levels may vary from standard lab reference ranges and are based on levels considered optimal by integrative and functional medicine practitioners.

Optimal level:*

- Fasting insulin: less than 8 uIU/mL

What it tells you:

- In a fasting state, your pancreas should not be pumping out a lot of insulin.
- Sleep deprivation or sleep apnea can affect insulin levels, so be sure to get restorative sleep.
- If it's elevated, consider chromium supplements along with a soluble fiber supplement.

TSH (thyroid stimulating hormone) Test

What it measures:

- Marker of thyroid function.

Optimal level:*

- Less than 2.0

What it tells you:

- Thyroid dysfunction can be a barrier to achieving and maintaining healthy weight. If TSH is higher than 2.0, explore treatment options with your doctor. A complete thyroid panel should include: free T3, T4, antithyroglobulin, TPO (thyroid peroxidase) and reverse T3. To support thyroid function, consider dietary supplements such as a comprehensive multivitamin-mineral supplement.

Vitamin D (serum 25-OH vitamin D) Test

What it measures:

- Vitamin D levels in the blood.

Optimal level:*

- 32–80 ng/mL

What it tells you:

- Vitamin D is an important fat-soluble vitamin with multiple functions, so maintaining healthy levels is essential. Vitamin D levels can be inhibited by gut dysfunction and excess body fat. Bring your levels into normal range with prudent sun exposure and vitamin D supplementation.

Serum Homocysteine Test

What it measures:

- Homocysteine is an amino acid that's important to vascular health and influenced by genetics.

Optimal level:*

- 4–10 umol/L

What it tells you:

- High levels of homocysteine can be due to impaired B-vitamin metabolism and absorption, so supplementing with B vitamins might be considered.
- Discuss family heart health history with your doctor, who may recommend additional tests.

Comprehensive Lipid Panel

What it measures:

- Total cholesterol; direct low-density lipoprotein, or LDL; high-density lipoprotein, or HDL; triglycerides; Lp(a); apo A-1 and apo B; lipoprotein particle number and size.

Optimal level:*

- Direct LDL: less than 100 mg/dL
- HDL: more than 60 mg/dL
- Triglycerides: less than 100 mg/dL

- TG:HDL ratio: less than 2
- Lp(a): less than 20 mg/dL
- LDL particle number: less than 1,000

What it tells you:

- When lipoprotein levels are included with the standard lipid measurements, more meaningful information is provided to make clinical decisions.
- Triglycerides are an independent cardiovascular risk factor for women; evaluating TG:HDL ratio and lipoprotein levels with particle size is most meaningful.
- There are also other biomarkers to determine risk, such as oxidized LDL.
- Consider soluble fiber as a first-line therapy and other possible supplements such as niacin, CoQ10, fish oils, red yeast rice, etc.

The Swift Supplement Prescription

The Swift supplement prescription is a collection of the nutraceuticals (another name for dietary supplements) that I have found most effective for helping to rebalance the digestive tract and supporting healthy weight management. I'll include a brief overview with recommended dosages, along with some caveats and considerations. This will give you the lay of the land, but it's not a substitute for the personal advice you receive from your health care provider. Before we jump in, take a close look at the sidebar on supplement "rules of the road," below.

SUPPLEMENT RULES OF THE ROAD

1. *Be informed.* As a clinical nutritionist, keeping up with the latest in dietary supplements is a monumental task, which is why I subscribe to the Natural Medicines Comprehensive Database (naturaldatabase .therapeuticresearch.com), an unbiased, scientific database on natural products. WebMD (http://www.webmd.com/vitamins-supplements/default.aspx) provides a handy layperson's guide. The most reliable watchdog on the Web is Consumer Lab (consumerlab.com), which periodically reviews natural products in the marketplace and does its own independent testing of ingredients. This site also has an informative Natural and Alternative Treatments encyclopedia that includes valuable facts on each product. The University of Maryland's Center for Integrative Medicine's Web site covering supplements is a font of well-organized information: http://www.compmed.umm.edu/resources_websites.asp. And the National Institutes of Health's Office of Dietary Supplements (http://ods.od.nih.gov/) can also give you the scoop on supplements with its handy fact sheets. I also encourage you to visit IntegrativeRD.org to find a registered dietitian/nutritionist in your area who can assess your individual needs and personalize your supplement prescription.

2. *Ask questions.* As you're doing your Web research, seek out the answers to the most important questions. For instance: Is a particular supplement "contraindicated" (don't take it!) for certain groups of people—pregnant women, children, people taking certain medications, people facing an upcoming surgery? Do the intended benefits seem to justify the known risks? Does the supplement have good evidence for safety? What are reasonably foreseeable side effects (for instance, gas and bloating)? What would be considered "adverse effects" (for instance, hives or high blood pressure)? Check out the FDA Web site that logs reported problems with supplements: http://www.fda.gov/Food/DietarySupplements/ReportAdverseEvent/.

3. *Evaluate the evidence as best you can.* Dig into the supporting research to see if the supplement studies were done in humans, in animals or in cell cultures. Understand that it's a big leap from animals to humans, an even bigger one from cell cultures to the human body. Are the doses used in the studies comparable to the dose recommended on the label? Is there any reliable evidence that supports the value of a supplement that comes from a source other than the company that makes or markets it?

4. *Choose wisely.* Study the labels! Get familiar with the ingredients and

fillers in a supplement so that you can avoid common allergens such as gluten, dairy, soy, corn or nuts if you have a problem with one or more of them. Some companies have started to avoid GMO ingredients and will tell you so on the label, which is a plus. A major concern is contamination with ingredients not listed on the labels and with outright toxins, including heavy metals. While this is a special concern with herbal supplements from China and India, in 2013 a major academic study found that a majority of North American herbal supplements it tested contained unlabeled "mystery" ingredients, some of them toxic. Go online to flag down any safety alerts: forewarned is forearmed. ConsumerLab.com subscribers have access to a list of supplements that passed its quality, purity and identity tests.

5. *Start "slow and low."* I like to start with one new supplement at a time and at the lowest most effective dose, based on the typical dose in studies. For example, if zinc sulfate has been studied for treating gastric ulcers at 200 mg three times daily then I recommend starting at 200 mg and gradually upping the dose from there. Wait and observe over a period of at least three days before increasing the dose or starting another supplement, in the event there is an adverse reaction.

6. *Observe and reevaluate.* When I recommend a supplement, I advise my clients to check in with me during the first one to two weeks to let me know how they are tolerating it (and sooner if they are not!). After that, ongoing monitoring and evaluation is essential, including changes in signs and symptoms and laboratory data. An effect from a supplement may show up in a few days or take up to three to six months.

I've grouped the supplements that I commonly use with clients into three groups: Weight Loss and Digestive Health; Digestive Health; Overall Health.

Weight Loss and Digestive Health

Fiber Supplements

It's certainly a seductive idea: weight loss in a pill! Both pharmaceutical and nutraceutical companies pursue it like the holy grail, and why not? Consumers desperate to lose weight are spending billions of dollars annually on weight-loss products. However, the academic researchers who have looked at these products have been underwhelmed. For instance, a 2009 study in the *World Journal of Gastroenterology* reanalyzed seventy-seven studies on weight-loss aids and concluded, "lifestyle modification is still the safest and efficacious method of inducing a persistent weight loss."

I'll endorse that in a heartbeat! (And remember, by "lifestyle modification," they're including diet.) But the evidence that a select few types of supplements can enhance weight loss has gotten a lot stronger in the past few years. Number one on my list of nutraceutical allies are fiber supplements. A more recent review of dietary supplements and weight management found that these fiber supplements—psyllium, for instance—could potentially play a valuable supporting role, mostly by suppressing appetite.

This dovetails with my clinical experience. The vast majority of my clients don't need fiber supplements to manage their hunger—the meal plans and the recipes that you'll find in the Swift Diet take care of that. I'm much more likely to recommend a fiber product for digestive health— they're a great natural way to address elimination problems (constipation or diarrhea). But for some weight-loss clients, hunger *is* an issue. They'll come to me and say, "I'm desperate; I need a supplement!" I suggest that they take a fiber supplement before meals along with a large glass of water. These supplements are not a magic bullet. They can have side effects; for instance, increasing gas and bloating and generally gumming up the works if you're not careful to drink plenty of fluids. But for the client at her wit's end, they can provide an extra, and relatively inexpensive, push that sometimes makes a big difference.

Recall that in previous chapters we learned that plant foods contain fermentable fibers, prebiotic fibers that support gut health and weight loss, thanks to their beneficial effect on the gut microbiome. The fiber supplements that we're talking about here have a preponderance of insoluble fibers that pass through the system more quickly, within a day or so. Because fiber is always a matrix of different subtypes, these supplements likely have a mildly beneficial prebiotic effect as well, if nothing on the order of a serving of asparagus. But the major payoff is the appetite suppression—the stuff takes up a lot of room in the gut—and the enhancement of regularity. These supplements also bind with excess cholesterol and excrete it out of the system, lowering blood cholesterol and, by slowing down digestion, keeping blood sugar levels stable. The type of fiber supplement that you choose depends on the outcome you are hoping to achieve, something you'll want to discuss with your health care provider. The following list describes some common types of fiber supplements that I use most often in my practice.

Acacia fiber

Derived from the acacia senegal plant, acacia fiber is also known as gum acacia or gum arabic.

Benefit: Soluble fiber is a bulking agent; it can be used for constipation and to help with passage of complete bowel movements.

Favorite Brand: Renew Life Organic Clear Fiber

Psyllium seed husk

Derived from the plant *Plantago ovata*, also known as psyllium, ispaghula or isabgol.

Benefit: Partially fermentable (70 percent soluble); bulk-forming and helpful to improve and maintain GI motility; also useful in blood sugar and cholesterol management.

Favorite Brands: Frontier Natural Products Organic Psyllium Husk, whole or powdered; Konsyl Original Formula

Konjac root (glucomannan)

A component of the cell walls of the konjac plant, a water-soluble fiber.

Benefit: Useful for lowering cholesterol and blood sugar; may also help with constipation and weight loss.

Favorite Brand: PGX Natural Factors

Modified Citrus Pectin and PectaSol

A form of pectin found in many fruits and vegetables, especially in the peel of citrus fruits, apples and plums.

Benefit: Form of soluble fiber that is more easily absorbed in the digestive tract, which may help with reducing diarrhea, reducing cholesterol levels and increasing excretion of toxic metals (for example, mercury, lead and arsenic) in the body.

Favorite Brands: EcoNugenics PectaSol-C Modified Citrus Pectin; NutriCology Modified Citrus Pectin

"Mixed" Fiber Formulas

A mix of different fiber ingredients; some of these products may also contain herbal ingredients (such as prune, apple, inulin, oat bran, agar, guar gum, etc.)

Benefit: Varies with the type of product selected and can be used to manage weight, blood sugar, cholesterol and GI symptoms.

Favorite Brands: Metagenics MetaFiber; Thorne MediBulk; Garden of Life Raw Fiber

Troubleshooting

- Look for fiber supplement products that are free of common allergens, food colorings and additives.
- Fiber supplements should be taken with a large glass of water, at least

10 to 12 ounces. It is important to stay well hydrated when using fiber supplements, especially at the higher dosages.

- Start with the lowest dose per product guidelines and gradually increase over time to achieve the desired effect.
- Side effects may include bloating, diarrhea and gas, especially when starting fiber supplements. If symptoms worsen while taking a fiber supplement, this may be due to an intolerance to oligosaccharide, one of the FODMAP elements.
- Be aware that fiber supplements can bind with many medications, vitamins and minerals and inhibit their absorption. Therefore, take one hour before or two hours after medications and other supplements.
- Be sure to check with your doctor, pharmacist or dietitian/nutritionist about known interactions, contraindications and cautions when using fiber supplements.

Probiotics

Like fiber supplements, probiotics can do double duty, enhancing both digestive health and weight loss. Professor Angelo Tremblay, a world leader in obesity research and the lead author of the Canadian probiotic study I talked about in Chapter 1, thinks that a significant part of the weight-loss effect comes from the probiotic's effect on the gut bacteria that influence the hormones that regulate appetite. The women on the probiotic supplements in his study lost more weight, he believes, because they were less hungry, so consequently they ate less. Another team of French researchers from the University of Rouen takes this idea further. They speculate that the microbiome may directly influence our food preferences. In effect, bad bacteria stimulate our appetite for the bad food that feed *them* and make *us* fat. The good bacteria, the kind helped by the probiotics, push our appetite in the opposite direction, toward nutritious, high-fiber foods. It does make you wonder who's in charge here.

So we have a glimpse of a fast-approaching future where we'll be able to confidently leverage the power of the microbiome for weight loss. Clearly, we're still in the experimental stage now. What are the best weight-loss-promoting bacterial strains? How best to combine them? These questions are being studied with some urgency, since probiotics look to deliver weight-loss enhancement with minimal side effects, compared to popular and potentially dangerous over-the-counter or pharmaceutical products that act as stimulants and rev up the central nervous system or cause malabsorption of important nutrients. But probiotics have been more extensively studied for digestive health, and I'm more likely to recommend them to my clients for that reason. If you're taking probiotics to rebuild your gut bacteria after a course of antibiotics or to address symptoms of gut upset and you're able to track a weight-loss effect, consider yourself part of a discovery process at the frontiers of scientific weight management!

Let's review. The official definition of a probiotic supplement is a "product that contains live microorganisms and when taken in adequate amounts confers a health benefit to the host." In Chapter 4, you learned about nourishing your digestive tract with traditional fermented foods, the original food-sourced probiotic therapy! On the supplement front there is evidence supporting the benefit of probiotics for a wide range of gut-related symptoms and disorders, such as food allergies, constipation, diarrhea, irritable and inflammatory bowel disease (ulcerative colitis and Crohn's). In addition, probiotics show promise in the treatment of a much broader constellation of conditions including allergies, asthma, autism, high cholesterol, genitourinary infections and rheumatoid arthritis. Ongoing research is looking at the role of "synbiotics," a combined formula containing a prebiotic such as inulin and a probiotic or probiotic mix of microorganisms. You may need to experiment with different types of probiotics to find the right match for your digestive tract.

I have included a list on the next page that outlines the main clinical benefits of some common probiotic products. In addition to these products, a number of dietary supplement companies have their own probiotic lines.

Popular Probiotic Products

CULTURELLE

Microorganism strain(s): *Lactobacillus casei* subsp. *rhamnosus* GG

Clinical benefit: Prevents rotavirus-related diarrhea in children; GI disorders in children

FLORASTOR

Microorganism strain(s): *Saccharomyces boulardii* (a probiotic yeast)

Clinical benefit: For travelers and antibiotic-associated diarrhea; IBS and IBD, Crohn's; recurrent *C. difficile* infection

ALIGN

Microorganism strain(s): *Bifidobacterium infantis* 35624

Clinical benefit: Supports healthy digestive system

BIO-K+

Microorganism strain(s): *Lactobacillus acidophilus* CL1285 and *Lactobacillus casei* LBC80R

Clinical benefit: For general digestive health

VSL#3

Microorganism strain(s): 4 strains of lactobacillus (*L. casei*, *L. plantarum*, *L. acidophilus*, *L. delbrueckii* subsp. *Bulgaricus*); 3 strains of bifidobacterium (*B. longum*, *B. breve*, *B. infantis*), 1 strain of *Streptococcus salivarius* subsp. *thermophilus*

Clinical benefit: For treatment of irritable bowel syndrome (IBS) and inflammatory bowel disease (IBD); pouchitis

Troubleshooting

- For general health purposes, I recommend a high-quality, broad-spectrum probiotic that contains a variety of lactobacilli and bifido-bacteria strains.
- When starting a probiotic, begin with a dose supplying approximately 1 to 10 billion CFU (colony forming units). You can also consider taking the probiotic in divided doses (e.g., 5 billion CFU twice daily).
- There is inadequate research on the best time to take probiotics; however, many probiotic scientists I have consulted recommend taking them with food.
- Take note of the recommended storage conditions; some probiotics require refrigeration. They should have an expiration date.
- Probiotics could possibly make some health problems worse; for example, SIBO, small intestinal overgrowth. Again, more research is needed. Be sure to check with your health care provider about any contraindications to taking probiotics—for example, cancer therapies—and any known possible drug interactions. Discuss how to space out taking medications (antibiotics, for instance) and probiotic supplements.
- The jury is still out on identifying the best probiotic or probiotic mix for various health conditions. Research will continue to identify the ways in which probiotics promote intestinal healing, improve immunity, reduce inflammation and prevent and treat GI disorders and the specific strains and dosages that will help.

Swift Notes

- Keep in mind that some people do not tolerate any form of dairy, including probiotic supplements that are dairy based. Fortunately, there are many probiotics that are suitable alternatives.
- Research is needed to determine if, once started, probiotics should be taken for the long term. The research suggests that the beneficial bac-

teria may not permanently take up residence in the gut, so a regular dose of probiotics from food or supplements is likely needed.

- Stay abreast of product evaluations in the marketplace at consumerlab .com and ongoing developments at International Scientific Association for Probiotics and Prebiotics, isaap.com.

Digestive Health

Betaine Hydrochloride (Betaine HCL/Trimethylglycine)

This is a manufactured form of hydrochloric acid that, when taken as a supplement, increases the amount of this digestive acid working in the stomach. Why would we want that? Don't people take over-the-counter and prescription drugs to reduce the stomach acid that causes gastric reflux? The truth is, while popping a pill to tamp down heartburn after an occasional over-spicy meal isn't a federal offense, the long-term use of acid-suppression drugs to deal with chronic stomach irritation is a misguided strategy. As we age, the stomach produces less hydrochloric acid, which we need for a host of reasons: it maintains the acid environment in the gut, which keeps harmful bacteria and other pathogens at bay; it triggers the release of pepsin and other enzymes necessary for digestion, especially of protein; it aids with the digestion and absorption of nutrients—so insufficient hydrochloric acid sets the stage for serious nutrient deficiencies in vitamin B_{12}, magnesium, iron, calcium and zinc.

Dosages: Betaine HCL capsules vary in dose. Start with one capsule of 350 mg Betaine HCL at the beginning of each meal. Monitor and gradually increase to effective dosage.

Troubleshooting

- Do not take HCL if you have an active ulcer, esophagitis or gastritis!
- HCL might also cause heartburn, so monitor carefully and discontinue if you have any symptoms.
- There are a number of combination formulas that contain Betaine

HCL plus other enzymes such as pepsin along with gentian bitters or other botanicals that can be helpful for digestive support.

Swift Notes: I consider HCL adequacy in all of my patients over fifty and especially those with chronic symptoms of deficiency such as bloating, belching, undigested food in stools and skin disorders. I continue to be amazed how often this simple supplement strategy pays dividends. But it often requires a lot of convincing, since most people think the problems they have are due to excess, not insufficient, stomach acid!

Deglycyrrhizinated Licorice (DGL)

DGL soothes the digestive system by promoting the body's production of mucus that coats the stomach and intestine, and it can be safely used for treating gastroesophageal reflux (GERD), canker sores and gastritis. Licorice root (*Glycyrrhiza glabra*) has been used in both Eastern and Western medicine for thousands of years to treat a variety of disorders, ranging from asthma to liver disease. But DGL is a special type that has had the glycyrrhizin removed (hence "deglycyrrhizinated"), a compound that can cause serious side effects, such as elevated blood pressure, lowered blood potassium (hypokalemia) and edema. Sometimes referred to as the "lining tamer," DGL is available in both capsules and lozenges.

Dosage: DGL lozenge (extract 4:1): Chew 300 to 400 mg, two to three times daily, ten to twenty minutes before meals.

Troubleshooting

- Be sure to check your product carefully to ensure it is DGL, not pure licorice root.
- Clinical trials demonstrating DGL's long-term effectiveness and ongoing safety need to be conducted.

Swift Note: I recommend DGL on a short-term basis to help clients troubled by heartburn and reflux, often to taper off medications, in consultation with their physician. I usually recommend a thirty-day trial and then reevaluate based on the response—it doesn't work for everybody. Some clients will use a DGL lozenge only on occasion, for the occasional gastric flare-up.

Digestive Enzymes

The digestive tract secretes a number of enzymes that help break down food into smaller molecules so that it can be more easily digested and eventually absorbed. That is, except when the body happens not to have enough of a particular necessary enzyme. If you're lactose intolerant, for example, you don't have enough of the lactase enzyme to break down the milk sugars in dairy and the result is gas, bloating and abdominal discomfort. As we discussed in Chapter 3, a number of foods can provoke these kinds of reactions, but fortunately we can supplement our body's natural enzyme supply to lessen, sometimes even get rid of, these adverse food reactions.

The enzyme supplements I usually recommend to my clients come from plant sources—bromelain from pineapple, papain from papaya, ficain from fig and actinidin from kiwi, to name a few. But enzymes derived from animal and microbial sources have their place for certain problems. In general, fat maldigestion can be improved with lipase supplementation—lipases are responsible for the breakdown of lipids. Proteases or proteolytic enzymes help break down protein foods. Specific proteases can be helpful in reducing the symptoms associated with dairy and wheat intolerances. Researchers are looking at supplemental enzymes that contain dipeptidyl peptidase IV (DPP-IV), which may have therapeutic value in breaking down gluten and casein, a milk protein.

Gut-related disorders and adverse food reactions have been stealthily on the rise, and the systemic inflammation caused by leaky gut is a prime suspect. Histamine intolerance is an increasingly recognized sensitivity to a common chemical found in a wide range of foods, including alcohol, fish, aged cheeses and egg whites, and it's produced by our bodies as well. The enzyme that breaks down histamine is called diamine oxidase (DAO), also made by our bodies. In addition to modifying your diet to lower the histamine load, DAO enzyme supplementation can also be helpful.

Although we have a lot more to learn about digestive enzymes and their effects on health, a broad-spectrum or multienzyme product can be of benefit in a wide range of gut-related disorders.

Dosages: Plant-based enzymes: Start with one capsule or tablet at the beginning of a meal or snack. This can be increased to two caps or tablets per meal.

Troubleshooting

- These supplements should not be taken by people with an active ulcer, pancreatitis, gastritis or history of elevated amylase.
- Be sure your enzyme formula has enzyme activities based on Food Chemical Codex (FCC) and United States Pharmacopeia (USP) standards.
- Do not take enzymes with hot beverages because this might decrease the enzyme activity. Improvements are generally seen immediately, but may take several days or weeks. You might notice a slight increase in bowel movement frequency and gas when beginning digestive enzymes.
- Some forms of enzymes may interfere with medications, so be sure to check with your health care provider.

Swift Notes: Some enzyme formulas might also contain botanicals such as quercetin, a bioflavonoid that can tamp down the response to environmental allergens.

Ginger (*Zingiber officinale*)

Ginger is probably best known for its use as a motion sickness aid, but it's also shown promise for treating osteoarthritis, vertigo, dysmenorrhea, morning sickness and a wide range of gastrointestinal symptoms. Different chemical compounds are responsible for ginger's gut-protective effects.

Some reduce inflammation in the gastrointestinal tract; some calm down the nervous system and may enhance gut motility, and hence regularity. Ginger may also have cholesterol- and blood-sugar-lowering effects, and it is being looked at as a complementary therapy for weight management.

Dosage: The dose depends on the condition being treated. For gastro-protective effects, I usually recommend starting with 250 mg taken three times daily and increase gradually up to 1 to 2 grams daily.

Troubleshooting: Because ginger has blood-thinning (antiplatelet) effects, it can increase the risk of bleeding in some people, although I have rarely encountered this in practice. A number of other dietary supplements can do something similar—omega-3 fatty acids, garlic, angelica, clove, gingko, Panax ginseng, red clover, turmeric—so review with your health care provider any cumulative effects and any potential ginger–prescription medication interactions.

Swift Note: There are certainly other ways to get ginger besides supplements! Brew some strong ginger tea, add freshly grated or dried ginger to your favorite recipes, including salad dressings, soups, stews and main dishes. But it takes a lot of fresh ginger to have a therapeutic effect, so when I want a greater digestive healing boost for an irritable bowel, I recommend ginger capsules.

Peppermint (*Mentha piperita*)

Peppermint contains menthol, a volatile oil and a popular ingredient in gum, teas, toothpaste, and cosmetics. It's a calming agent for the skin and gastrointestinal tract since it relaxes the muscles of the stomach and improves the flow of bile, which helps with fat digestion. Several studies have shown that enteric-coated peppermint capsules can effectively treat IBS symptoms such as bloating, gas, pain and diarrhea. So, peppermint is often my first "go to" supplement for IBS.

Dosage: For IBS, use enteric-coated peppermint capsules, 0.2 to 0.4 ml, three times a day, with food.

Troubleshooting

- Because it relaxes the "doorway" or sphincter muscle between the stomach and esophagus, peppermint can also aggravate reflux and should not be used if someone has been diagnosed with GERD or hiatal hernia.
- Peppermint may interact with some medications, especially acid-reducing drugs, so be sure to take it at least two hours before or after any antacids.
- Some peppermint products also contain a blend of herbal ingredients such as thyme, ginger, fennel or rosemary oil. Iberogast (STW 5, Medical Futures, Inc.) contains a specific combination of peppermint leaf plus clown's mustard plant, German chamomile, caraway, licorice, milk thistle, angelica, celandine and lemon balm. A number of studies have demonstrated that it's an effective herbal for functional dyspepsia and IBS and it's well tolerated for long-term treatment. The typical dosage of Igerogast is 1 ml three times daily.

Swift Note: I have worked with many clients who suffered from IBS for years, unaware that peppermint might be helpful. One of my patients wasn't open to taking supplements but was willing to try peppermint tea. She started sipping on peppermint tea (three teabags per cup!) between meals, and after a few weeks she reported that she was hooked on it—she felt it helped keep her gas and bloating symptoms under control. Some medical practitioners also treat digestive complaints by rubbing a few drops of peppermint oil on the belly, counterclockwise and down in the direction of the transverse and descending colon to help stool movement and elimination. I know a few who swear by it!

Overall Health

Magnesium

Magnesium is a magnificent mineral that actively participates in hundreds of biochemical reactions that impact our mood, muscles, nerves, bones, blood sugar, digestive health, weight and even our ability to detoxify! Although it is widely distributed in many plant foods, especially dark greens, beans, legumes, nuts and seeds, our soils may not be as rich in this vital mineral as they used to be. Most people just don't get enough. And too much alcohol, prolonged stress and a number of medications, including oral contraceptive agents, lower magnesium levels. It's also important to note that many medical conditions upset magnesium balance, especially gut disorders such as irritable bowel syndrome, liver disease (cirrhosis) and ulcerative colitis. Symptoms of magnesium deficiency are diverse and can include irritability, anxiety, depression, fibromyalgia, chronic fatigue, muscle spasms and weakness, migraines, restless leg syndrome (RLS), low blood pressure, abnormal heart rhythms, poor nail growth, nausea, constipation and sleep problems. Take note of that last one. A magnesium supplement can make a great sleep aid. No knockout pill, no hangover, just a relaxing way to encourage and enhance sleep.

Dosage: The type and dosage of magnesium depends on the condition being treated, so I'm focusing on just a few gut-related symptoms here.

Constipation: Magnesium citrate, start with 250 mg/day with food and increase up to 6,000 mg/day until good bowel function resumes.

To improve magnesium status: Magnesium glycinate, 125 to 250 mg per day with food

Sleep: Magnesium glycinate, 125 to 250 mg at bedtime

Troubleshooting

- This multifaceted mineral has many potential interactions with other nutrients, herbs, lab tests and medications, so it's important to check with your health care provider to fine-tune your supplementation.
- Magnesium supplements can cause loose bowels, so decrease the dose to a level your bowels can easily tolerate.

Swift Note: For years, I practiced as a renal dietitian, and the kidney remains near and dear to me. Anyone with reduced kidney function should check with their physician *before* using magnesium supplements, due to an increased risk of elevating your blood magnesium level (hypermagnesemia).

Omega-3 Fatty Acids

As we discussed in Chapter 4, the omega-3s, one type of polyunsaturated fatty acids (PUFAs), are *essential* fatty acids. You've got to get them from food sources, and because a lot of people don't eat much fish, the richest source, there's a case to be made for fish oil supplements. As with any supplement, I tailor my fish oil recommendation to the individual. If you're eating two or three servings of fish a week, supplements may not be necessary. But let's say you're not a fish eater. Or you're showing signs of inflammation that might show up on the lab test for C-reactive protein or in symptoms that might range from gut disorders to joint and skin problems. Then the omega-3s can be a powerful tool in your supplement toolbox. While the research record isn't as bulletproof as we once thought, there's still very good evidence for them as anti-inflammatory agents that support immune, cardiovascular, joint and brain health. In other studies, they show promise helping to treat inflammatory bowel disease, hypertriglyceridemia (high triglyceride levels), high blood pressure and rheumatoid arthritis and supporting healthy infant development in pregnancy.

Supplements can be manufactured from animals (fish) or plants (seed oils, algal sources). Fish oils contain the preferred and "preformed" omega-

3s (EPA and DHA), while the body must convert the plant omega-3 (ALA) into EPA and DHA, which it does very inefficiently.

There are two main groups of omega-3 fatty acid supplements:

Fish Oil

- EPA (eicosapentaenoic acid) and DHA (docosahexaenoic acid) (anchovy, menhaden, salmon, krill [shrimplike crustacean], squid/calamari).
- Fish oils come in capsules or as liquid supplements and contain both EPA and DHA.
- One gram of fish oil usually contains 180 mg EPA and 120 mg DHA.
- Cod liver oil also contains EPA and DHA. Cod liver oil and fish oils are not the same thing because cod liver oil, extracted from the livers of cod, provides additional fat-soluble vitamins A and D.

Plant Seed Oils

- Alpha-linolenic acid (ALA) from flax, hemp, and chia seed oils. ALA is converted to DHA or EPA, but only in minimal amounts.

Dosage: A wide range of dosages are used, depending on the condition. I usually recommend between 1,000 and 2,000 mg per day for non-fish eaters, taken at a meal that includes some healthy fat. Higher doses of fish oils in the range of 2 to 10 grams per day may be recommended based on the individual's health status and dietary intake. For vegans, 400 to 600 mg a day of algae-based DHA supplements in combination with nuts and seeds is a workable strategy.

Troubleshooting

- It is important to purchase a reputable brand of fish oils to obtain a product that meets a high standard of freshness and purity and is free of contaminants. A few of my favorite brands are Carlson, Kirkland, Nordic Naturals and Metagenics.
- Omega-3 fish oil supplements may have some unpleasant side effects, such as fishy taste, belching, nausea and loose stools. Enteric coated

products are designed to help avoid "fish burp" but may cost a bit more than regular products.

- Although it's rare, fish oils may increase the risk of bleeding in some individuals. Be informed if you're taking any medications or other supplements that increase your risk.
- Omega-3 supplements are also made from krill oil, but because krill is a major food source for aquatic animals, such as whales, seals and penguins, environmental concerns have been raised.

Swift Note

- A lab test that measures fatty acids in the blood can be helpful to tailor fatty acid supplement recommendations.
- Gamma-linolenic acid (GLA) is an omega-6 fatty acid found in evening primrose, black currant and borage oils. I have found GLA supplements to be helpful for individuals with breast tenderness, eczema, psoriasis and arthritis. Some omega-3 supplements contain GLA, and your health care provider can guide you as to the best fatty acid supplement to meet your needs.

Vitamin D

Vitamin D is the sunshine vitamin—our bodies are able to synthesize it from sunshine in large amounts during the warm-weather months. And we can get it in smaller amounts from food sources and, if that's not sufficient, in supplement form. All told, it's a multitasking fat-soluble vitamin involved in immunity, bone health, cardiovascular health, cancer prevention, mood, depression, neurological disorders such as multiple sclerosis (MS) and even obesity—a busy hormone and micronutrient! Research continues to uncover the mechanisms by which this critical nutrient affects so many things beyond bone health and even decreases the overall death rate ("all-cause mortality"). But as a clinician, I can tell you that vitamin D supplements, for people with chronically low D levels, can make a major difference in their health status. Clients will sometimes tell me they feel more energetic; they'll say they're amazed how few winter colds they caught.

Vitamins and minerals "cross-talk," so we have to consider D's balance within the entire nutrient symphony. The recommended allowance for vitamin D established by the Food and Nutrition Board of the Institute of Medicine is 600 to 800 IUs per day for adults. A "tolerable upper limit" has been established at 4,000 IUs. I think the best advice is to "test, don't guess." Most research suggests that achieving a serum 25-OH vitamin D level of greater than 20 ng/mL is adequate. However, many integrative doctors suggest an optimal range of 32 to 80 ng/mL.

There are two dietary forms of vitamin D: ergocalciferol (vitamin D_2) and cholecalciferol (vitamin D_3). Vitamin D is found naturally in foods such as fatty fish (salmon, mackerel, tuna, sardines, herring); cod liver oil and eggs. It's also added to fortified foods such as dairy (milk, yogurt, cheese, etc.), nondairy beverages (almond, soy, etc.), grain products (cereals) and other functional foods such as energy bars and drinks. Recently, white button mushrooms have been used to harvest vitamin D from UV light.

Dosage: The right dose should be based on achieving an optimal serum vitamin D level of *at least* 20 ng/mL. You should have your vitamin D level checked at least twice each year, in the spring and fall. If your level is low, start with 2,000 IUs vitamin D_3 (cholecalciferol) taken with a meal that has some healthy fat in it. Ask your doctor to recheck your level in three months to make sure you are in an optimal range. And be sun smart—"incidental" sunlight exposure for as little as ten to fifteen minutes per day can help improve your vitamin D status.

Troubleshooting

- Some people aren't as good at synthesizing vitamin D from sunlight— dark-skinned individuals, obese people and those who have undergone gastric bypass surgery—so they're at greater risk for developing vitamin D deficiency. Conversely, because D is fat soluble and can be stored in the body, some people by virtue of their genetics are *too* good at storage and are at greater risk for toxicity. So, have your blood levels checked and be on the lookout for symptoms of D overload like: a metallic taste in the mouth, increased thirst, bone pain, fatigue, itchy skin, muscle aches and pains, urinary frequency and gastrointestinal symptoms including nausea, vomiting, diarrhea and constipation.

- Vitamin D has the potential to interact with many medications such as cholesterol-lowering drugs, corticosteroids, seizure medications and others, so be sure to check with your health care provider if you are routinely taking any medications.
- Vitamin D supplementation is contraindicated in cases of pulmonary sarcoidosis and hyperparathyroidism.
- Stay tuned as the debate continues regarding the optimal level of vitamin D in the blood and the amount of vitamin D supplementation needed to achieve this level.
- Check out vitamindcouncil.org for research updates on this fascinating vitamin.

Swift Note: My mom had rickets, the classic vitamin D deficiency disease, when she was a toddler, so this vitamin has always intrigued me. And I'm happy to see an increase in the number of people who are having their D levels checked. A few years ago, when I asked large groups of health professionals if anyone had had their levels checked, only a few hands would go up. In the past couple of years, that's gone up to a third or more of the audience. That's progress, but not good enough, considering vitamin D's far-reaching effect on our health.

Zinc

Zinc can be a paradox. It's one of the most common mineral deficiencies in the Western diet, and low concentrations of it have been associated with elevated levels of fat in the blood, inflammation, insulin resistance and obesity. On the other hand, probably because it's been shown to be able to reduce the duration and severity of the common cold, some people overdo it with the supplementation. I had one patient who came to me for severe nausea and significant unintentional weight loss, convinced that she had cancer. When I discovered that between her multivitamin-mineral and her other supplements she was taking more than 150 mg of supplemental zinc daily, I told her to discontinue all supplements for a week. The following week she called me in tears. For the first time in over a year, she had no nausea and felt that she could eat again!

But in the proper amounts, we need zinc for the regulation of blood sugar and for myriad other body processes: vision, thyroid function, brain health, reproductive fitness, wound healing and immunity. Zinc has anti-oxidant properties and acts as a cellular guardian by scavenging harmful free radicals. Many conditions increase the body's need for zinc, including gastrointestinal disorders such as celiac disease, ulcerative colitis and Crohn's disease. When our bodies don't get enough zinc, the symptoms can be all over the map and include lack of taste and smell, depression, poor wound healing, hair loss, night blindness and skin changes such as acne, dermatitis and psoriasis.

Rich food sources of zinc include animal foods such as shellfish (especially oysters), red meat, poultry and cheese. It's also found in plant foods, including legumes like the soy foods tofu and miso, whole grains, greens and seeds (pumpkin, sesame and sunflower). However, the anti-nutrient phytate in plants can interfere with absorption of zinc. The Swift Diet offers the best of both worlds—limited amounts of animal protein and some fermented foods that help disarm the phytate and enhance the availability of minerals like zinc.

There are many different types of supplemental zinc available—lozenges, capsules, nasal sprays. Zinc sulfate is often the least expensive form but can cause stomach upset. I use zinc citrate to supplement dietary intake and use a special form of zinc called zinc carnosine as a healing agent for gastrointestinal symptoms including inflammation, dyspepsia and GERD.

Dosages: The dosage depends on the condition you are treating. For the common cold: at the first sign of symptoms, take a zinc lozenge, every two to three hours, up to 40 mg zinc daily. For general wellness, take zinc citrate, 15 mg daily. For digestive healing, zinc carnosine, 75 mg daily (17 to 18 mg elemental zinc/58 mg L-carnosine).

Troubleshooting: Like most vitamins and minerals, zinc interacts with other nutrients—too much zinc can cause a copper imbalance, for instance. Zinc also interacts with a number of medications, such as blood-pressure drugs, thiazide diuretics, antibiotics, chemotherapy agents and immuno-suppressant medications. Toxicity is also a potential concern at high doses.

Closing Thoughts

The dietary supplement industry is big business, and marketing claims are plentiful and enticing, especially to the person struggling with health issues. While this chapter isn't (and shouldn't be) a precise road map for using supplements to support digestive health and weight loss, I've given you some ideas that I hope will be useful on the journey you'll take with your personal health care provider.

Chapter 6

S: SUSTAINING PRACTICES

Beth

Beth is a hard-charging Manhattan publishing executive. When I first met her at Canyon Ranch, her routine was simply depleting. Dinner was takeout or going out with business associates to cocktail parties or restaurants—near-constant work-related socializing. She went to bed around midnight with a stack of spreadsheets and book manuscripts, so she didn't actually fall asleep until around two a.m. If iPads and smartphones had been around when I first started working with her, she would have gone to bed with them too—so many of my clients now glow in the dark as they catch up on the day's e-mails and Web surfing.

Beth admitted to me that her batteries were running down. Her weight was up, her energy was down and the usual middle-age warning lights were flashing—elevated cholesterol and blood pressure. While she was at the Ranch, she braved the scale and the number that came up got her attention. Still, she didn't deprive herself at mealtimes—the delicious, healthy cuisine was a big part of the draw. But eating at regular hours, going to bed earlier and being physically active in the morning—she loved the nature walks—had an effect after just a couple of days. She was hungry for breakfast in the morn-

ing, getting back in tune with her body's natural rhythms. When we checked in on the last day of her five-day stay, she was surprised that she had dropped four pounds, something she'd long written off as impossible.

When I worked with Beth after her stay, we made some permanent changes in her routine that paid off. When she went out in the evenings to social events, she alternated glasses of club soda with a splash of bitters with her usual wine, cutting down on the empty calories. I can't say Beth became an ardent home cook, but she held on to the concept of healthy portion size no matter where she was eating, and she ordered meals she never would have dreamed of ordering before—fish rather than steak; a side salad and vegetable instead of fries; fruit for dessert. And she joined a gym and had a personal trainer who made sure she stuck to her moderate exercise routine three times a week. She put down her work an hour before bedtime with rare exceptions, and turned to her wish list of novels she'd wanted to read for years! Nothing radical, nothing that pushed her too far outside of her comfort zone. The weight kept coming off and in less than two years she'd lost thirty-five pounds and had gotten a clean bill of health from her physician. Best of all, she has maintained her weight and health to this day, and I have no doubt into the future.

SELF-INQUIRY BOX

1. Do you go to bed with your iPad?
2. Do you sometimes feel like you're trapped on a speeding stress treadmill?
3. Have you ever been curious about trying out a mind-body practice like yoga or qigong?

n Chapter 2, we learned about how the mind and gut are connected and how everything from ideas and emotions to the timing of your meals can affect digestion and weight. In Chapters 3 and 4, we learned about the nuts and bolts of healthy eating and weight loss: which foods to eliminate or restrict; which foods nourish the body and promote healthy digestion and weight. Chapter 5 was devoted to supplements, how supplements can provide significant "value added," with probiotics in particular bringing us closer to an era of individually tailored "microbiomatic" health and weight loss.

So what's left? Chapter 6, "S: Sustaining Practices," is about everything else! It's about how you live most of your life. The everyday routines we develop, or fall back into, will, in large measure, determine whether we will continue to make smart eating choices and stay on the nourishing life course we've set for ourselves. You may recall that I ended Chapter 1 with the idea that successful weight loss and digestive health was about "digesting" your life as a whole.

Consider my client Beth, the high-powered New York City publishing executive. I began working with her before most of the new microbiome research was even dreamed of. Even if that research had been available to provide a nutritional blueprint, she was never going to be meticulous in her approach to cooking and eating. But just making some simple changes to reboot a manifestly unhealthy lifestyle, without pushing a meal plan that was more rigorous than her temperament would tolerate, made such a difference. In the Swift Diet, when we combine a healthy lifestyle with a mostly plant-food, mostly home-cooked diet that operates in sync with the microbiome, even bigger things are possible.

In 2012, I served on a panel that was convened by Lieutenant General Patricia Horoho, the U.S. Army surgeon general, to discuss a program she was spearheading to improve the health of our armed forces. Traditionally, army doctors were mostly concerned with patching up soldiers after combat. But Lieutenant General Horoho was facing a scenario where three out of four young Americans weren't even eligible for military service in large measure because of weight and medical issues. And so she was consulting a wide range of health care professionals to develop a program to get at the root of this rot. She called it "the Triad": sleep, exercise and nutrition. I think the army surgeon general picked her targets well.

In this chapter, I'm going to zero in on two major areas, sleep and exercise, which provide a lifestyle foundation for the eating plan that follows in the next chapter. Sleep, exercise and nutrition really do form an interlocking triad. Think about it. Good, sufficient sleep provides us with the physical energy required to do the exercise that revs up the metabolism and builds the lean muscle tissue that burns calories and promotes weight loss. It also contributes to the mental clarity and positive mood that we need to continue to make smart food choices. Bad, insufficient sleep? We're liable to slip into a groggy state of distraction that is a recipe for falling off the wagon. And insufficient sleep undoes us at the biochemical level as well. It drives up levels of our primary stress hormone, cortisol, which pumps up the body's production of insulin and drives cravings for sweets and fast-digesting carbs. In turn, regular exercise promotes a good night's sleep— when the body is tired, in a healthy way, the mind tends to shut off when we turn off the light at night. And especially for people who suffer from the common health problem of sleep apnea, losing weight can dramatically improve the quality of their sleep. The arrows connecting the three elements of the triad run in every direction you can imagine.

This isn't just for beginners. I have clients who are very successful at losing weight by following the diet changes I lay out and then eventually— it's the same for any woman on any diet—the progress will slow down or even halt, sometimes before they reach their personal goals. This is the plateau phase. That's when we need to reboot the lifestyle elements that are keeping you stuck at a weight that you're not happy with or suffering unpleasant (or worse) digestive symptoms. Beyond sleep and exercise, in the second half of this chapter we'll shift the focus inward, introducing some basics from two mind-body traditions, yoga and qigong. If improving your sleep and exercise was about getting your body in tune with the demands of the external world, this is about getting in tune with yourself!

At an obvious level, these mind-body techniques reduce stress and, as we discussed, calm the stress hormones that drive carb cravings. But in a subtler way, by encouraging us to focus all of our attention on synchroniz-ing the breath with a few relatively simple movements, they train us to block out the noise of everyday life and to be more present and in touch with ourselves as physical and even spiritual beings.

So, in a sense, we're finishing up the MENDS program where we began. In the M step we learned to bring attention to the way we eat and to begin to get a handle on the fears and anxieties that overstimulate the enteric nervous system. In this final section of the S chapter, we'll learn a few sys-tematic techniques to detach from those anxieties and lessen their grip.

Sleep: The Big Recharge

The more we learn about sleep, the more important it becomes. A brand-new avenue of research keys in on sleep as the brain's way to get rid of waste products in much the same way as the lymphatic system drains off waste from the rest of the body. It may well be that getting the seven to nine hours that sleep experts think most people need is the best way to protect against the excessive buildup of brain plaque that's implicated in neurodegenera-tive diseases like Alzheimer's. That's in addition to the established research linking poor sleep with increased rates of obesity, type 2 diabetes, high blood pressure, heart disease and premature death!

Indisputably, the lack of quality sleep drives weight gain and digestive problems, our main concerns here. The digestive part of the equation will probably come as no surprise. I imagine we've all had the experience of having to get up after only a few hours of sleep and discovering that our insides were in an uproar. Stress and sleep disruption have been found to affect gut motility—the speed at which the digestive system sends waste out of the body, sometimes too quickly, sometimes not fast enough, depending on the individual. The weight gain aspect is less obvious, more insidious, and women in particular seem more susceptible. In one recent in-patient study, subjects in a hospital setting were restricted to five hours of sleep for five nights, the equivalent of a stressed-out week of work deadlines and family responsibilities, and then allowed to sleep as long as they wanted for another five nights, up to nine hours a night. The men's weight fluctuated by only a small amount but the women gained on average about a pound on the sleep deprivation regimen and lost about half a pound with generous sleep.

So what's going on here? It won't surprise you by now that the gut microbiome is likely involved. Some interesting research showed that disrupting the sleep/wake cycle of mice increased the permeability or "leakiness" of their gut wall, which sets the stage for systemic inflammation and MicroObesity. Beyond the theoretical level, we know that lack of sleep is a body stressor that pumps up cortisol, associated with increased production of insulin, our fat-storage hormone, and, consequently, abdominal fat deposition. This makes sense in evolutionary terms. If you're trying to evade predators or survive long stretches without food, it's a handy thing to have a reserve energy supply around your middle. In our modern world, it's a disaster. These days, researchers consider chronic sleep deprivation a risk factor for insulin resistance, as in, what happens when the cells stop responding to all that extra insulin. Insulin resistance is the royal road to obesity, metabolic syndrome and, ultimately, type 2 diabetes.

The latest experimental work on sleep and weight gain goes beyond the hormonal explanations to look at how sleep deprivation, especially going to bed late, encourages gratuitous snacking. The researchers call it "emotional disinhibition." You can think of it as motive meeting opportunity. It's late at night, maybe you're zoned out watching TV and you reach for a cookie and then a few more, or a bag of chips. Or maybe you're hard at work on some important project and you feel the need for some extra calories to keep your brain fueled. You're right; the brain consumes about 70 percent of the glucose the body takes in, and the longer you're awake and the harder you're thinking, the more fuel you need. But night owls habitually overcompensate and eat more than what's required. Whatever the combination of physiology, psychology and environment—and it surely varies from person to person—the late-night lifestyle is a recipe for weight gain. Here's my plan to combat it.

SOS (SWIFT OPTIMAL SLEEP) PLAN

1. Take the TV out of the bedroom—the bed should be reserved for sleep and sex, both restorative. While you're at it, take the TV out of your kid's room. A recent Dartmouth study found that over the course of four years, adolescents who had TVs in their bedrooms gained about a pound a year more than their peers who didn't.

2. Set a bedtime that ensures at least seven hours of sleep and keep to it.

3. An hour or two before bedtime, cut yourself off—no more drinks, with or without alcohol. This cuts down on sleep-disturbing nocturnal visits to the bathroom. (And alcohol disrupts sleep patterns.)

4. Set a "snooze" alarm an hour before your bedtime and begin the slowing down/shutting down process: no more e-mails or TV and, emphatically, no iPad in bed, for two reasons. If you're working on a tablet, you're keeping your brain charged up, which works against falling asleep quickly and sleeping soundly. And even if you're reading an engaging and relaxing novel, the light rays emitted by these devices are just the right frequency to suppress the body's production of melatonin, which interferes with a good night's sleep at the hormonal level. A novel in bed is fine; just lose the iPad!

5. Keep the bedroom cool and dark after the lights go out.

6. Avoid "weekend jet lag." That is, get out of the pattern of sleep deprivation during the workweek, sleeping an hour or two less than you really need, and then trying to catch up on the weekend, sleeping in on Saturday and Sunday mornings. That has the effect of "resetting" your internal clock, equivalent to traveling two or three time zones away, and setting yourself up for a wretched "jet-lagged" Monday morning. Keep your weekend wake-up times within an hour or so of your workweek rise time. If you do need to play weekend sleep catch-up, take catnaps, not longer than twenty minutes a shot and not after 4 p.m.

Circadian Rhythms and Chronobiology

Sleep is actually part of a larger story about how our body is governed by its circadian rhythms. Think of these rhythms collectively as a timer in the cells of the body, synchronized to the patterns of light and dark over the course of a twenty-four-hour day. A new science has even grown up, chronobiology, that has discovered "clock genes" distributed throughout the cells of the body that in turn answer to a "master clock" located in the hypothalamus in the brain. These clocks help regulate a host of critical body processes, including the sleep/wake cycle, body temperature and the secretion of hormones. And when we depart too far from the way the system is genetically programmed, we pay a price. We're resilient, so an out-of-sorts week is unlikely to do us any permanent harm. But when we routinely take our meals at all hours of the day and night, the gut will likely register upset. (Yes, there is a "gut clock.") When we habitually keep strange hours and don't get enough quality sleep, we're at increased risk for everything from obesity to heart disease. This last one cuts especially close to home. My father was a shift worker in upstate New York and I strongly suspected the topsy-turvy hours he kept at his job contributed to his being overweight and then dying young from heart disease. The first paper I ever wrote as a nutrition undergrad in the seventies looked at this link between circadian rhythms and obesity.

Rhythm is such a powerful concept when we're thinking about how we want to address the day, not just for weight loss and digestive health, but for pleasure too! Most days should unfold with a predictable and reassuring rhythm, and meals are important rituals that are part of that flow.

The "Nature Cure"

Another big piece of that daily rhythm that's all too often ignored is spending time outdoors. At a purely physiological level, exposure to natural light fine-tunes our circadian rhythms and has a positive effect on mood. Researchers have discovered, for instance, that exposure to early-morning sun is an important natural check against depression and a potent natural antidepression therapy. Outdoor exercise is of course hugely beneficial—we'll get to that in the next section.

But there's something about being in nature itself, whether you're walking on a trail or just sitting on a park bench, that confers its own independent benefit. You don't have to book a trip to a national park. Any place where you share the space with some trees and plants and, if you're lucky, animals besides humans, will do the trick. The Harvard biologist E. O. Wilson coined the term *biophilia* to describe the human need to experience other species, and by extension the landscape they inhabit. Nature takes us out of ourselves and our preoccupations. Being in nature becomes a kind of meditation, whether we choose to think about it that way or not. Living in the Berkshires, I'm lucky enough to have easy access to a network of forests and hiking trails. My friend and coauthor Joe Hooper is a Manhattanite who credits short near-daily visits to Central Park with preserving the sanity of a longtime freelance writer.

I'm guessing most of you have had similar experiences even if you're not currently budgeting your time to make room for them. But I believe you should, even if it's just having lunch a few times a week in a local park or on the outdoor office picnic bench. The physical reality of nature is probably our best antidote for the unreality of a work life dominated by the computer, our downtime by TV and our social life (at any rate, our kids' social lives) by digital social media.

Richard Louv, author of *The Nature Principle*, dubs the effect "vitamin N," and it's supported scientific literature that has begun to measure its health *and* weight effects. In one study from the University of Essex in England, the same group of people took two walks of the same duration, through a country park and an indoor mall. While almost everyone in the group experienced a mood lift outdoors, 22 percent were *more* depressed after the mall walk! In a study in *American Journal of Preventive Medicine*, the researchers looked at the lives of over thirty-eight hundred inner-city children and found that, on average, the greener their neighborhoods, the lower the kids' body mass index!

"DIGITAL DETOX"

You don't have to go on a weeklong silent retreat to lessen your dependence on your digital devices (although that can be a wonderful thing to do). You can start by reclaiming weekends and vacations—remember when you used to have time for yourself or your family? Limit yourself to checking and responding to e-mails once or, at most, twice a day. As much as possible, don't respond to work e-mails on your time off—train the work world to respect your boundaries. And engage in activities that lend themselves to unplugging from work or the social buzz. Write in your journal, read that good book you couldn't find time for, go for a long walk in the woods or the park. My colleague, yoga teacher Jenne Young, suggests two ways of doing this: 1) Let your mind ramble along with your body; see where it and you go; 2) Make your stroll a walking meditation. Try to make yourself exquisitely sensitive to your surroundings and the feel of your body moving through them. Feel the air on your face, the ground underneath your feet. When you notice that you're thinking, return to these physical sensations.

Exercise: The Weight-Loss Edge

Exercise is, of course, a fantastic mood lifter, sleep enhancer and stress fighter. If you could patent it and put it in a pill, you'd have the most broadly effective and safest drug in the world. Studies have found exercise to be as good as or better than drugs in treating mild depression, and in a landmark 2013 study coauthored by Stanford epidemiologist Dr. John Ioannidis, exercise tested out about as well as drugs in the treatment of four common killers—heart disease, chronic heart failure, stroke and diabetes—without side effects.

When it comes to weight loss and digestive health, it's hard to overstate how good exercise can be for you. It may promote the growth of friendly bacteria in the gut. Getting moving certainly has the effect of getting the bowels moving, and constipation can set in motion all sorts of digestive problems you'd rather not deal with. When you're working out, you're doing a lot of things that the GI system appreciates:

- You're increasing the forces of gravity that are helping to send waste out of the system.
- You're stimulating the body's production of nitric oxide, which protects the mucous lining of the gut.
- You're also stimulating the body's lymphatic system, another waste removal system, which protects against bloating.

The pioneer in the field of digestive health and exercise—in the entire field of women and digestive health, actually—is Dr. Robynne Chutkan, a Georgetown University gastroenterologist and the founder of the Digestive Center for Women. Her book, *Gutbliss*, is a wonderful guide to the gut, and the nonprofit group she founded, GUTRUNNERS (gutrunners.com), works to bring attention to digestive health, with a special emphasis on exercise.

Most weight-loss veterans will tell you that losing weight is not nearly as challenging as keeping it from coming back. Here is where exercise really shines. One of my heroes in the obesity field, Dr. Rena Wing at Brown University, maintains a National Weight Control Registry of about ten thousand people, most of them women, who have lost a lot of weight (the average is seventy pounds) and kept it off for at least six years. The statistic that jumps out from this pool of weight-loss maintainers: they exercise, on average, the equivalent of a daily four-mile walk. If your weight-loss goals are more modest, you may not have to be quite as religious about exercise. But I and most of my clients are out there most days of the week doing something or some combination of things: walking, hiking, jogging, cycling, swimming laps, doing Pilates, Rollerblading, you name it.

An essential key is matching the person with the exercise that speaks to her.

Walking is perfect for the woman who hasn't been physically active for years, and swimming for the woman who is ready for something more physically demanding but who has joint issues. I've found Pilates often works well as one exercise component for women entering the perimeno-pausal years. Experiencing hormonally influenced weight gain, they want to regain control of their core. In the case of sports like jogging and cycling, it's often a question of recovering what you used to do and reclaiming it in the present.

My friend Reba Schecter, for twenty years the director of exercise physiology and physical therapy at Canyon Ranch in the Berkshires, puts it this way: "The best exercise is one that you enjoy doing. At any rate, you've got to enjoy it enough to keep doing it!"

Reba developed an exercise template for the Swift Diet that covers all the major fitness elements: cardio, strength, flexibility and balance. It provides the missing ingredient for those of us who know we need an exercise routine to supplement our weight-loss program but don't currently have one: structure. The program is self-paced, but you'll want to begin with some professional guidance. First, see your doctor and make sure that you don't have medical issues that would stand in the way of an exercise program that increases in intensity. Then consult with a physical therapist or an exercise physiologist for a session or two to go over any muscle and joint issues that need to be addressed. If you've been out of the game for a while, they'll provide a reintroduction to some exercise and exercise equipment basics. Then, if you choose, you're on your own. Or, if your schedule and finances permit, you might work with a knowledgeable trainer, either at a gym or at your house. For those of us whose motivation is a little shaky at the outset, this can be a great way to go.

The Cardio Burn

Let's tackle the elements in Reba's template, one at a time. Cardio is the most important. The endurance work is where you're going to get the steady calorie burn and what you're going to devote the most time to every week. It's mostly in the aerobic range; in other words, done at a comfortable pace where you can still carry on a conversation. Which activity you choose for the cardio work is up to you. It could be walking or jogging or cycling or, if you have access to a pool, swimming or pool aerobics. If you happen to live near a body of water bigger than a pool, kayaking or sculling is on the menu. The cardio machines at the gym are also fine, as is a vigorous sport like tennis (singles, not doubles). Mix and match as you see fit. The prescription is thirty minutes a day of cardio, done five to seven days a week. If you can do the routine every day without feeling washed out, do it; you'll reach your weight-loss goals that much faster. If you find yourself craving a rest day or two a week, take them. However, and this is a big however, if you suffer from a chronic pain or chronic fatigue syndrome, go much more cautiously. Exercise is therapeutic here, but in smaller doses. Work out every other day and carefully monitor how you're feeling. At the first sign of worsening symptoms, dial it back. Be sensitive to how much your body can and wants to handle. If at first you need to spread the thirty minutes out into two or three increments over the course of the day, that's fine.

As you'll see in Reba's list, this is a graduated program that gets more challenging as it progresses over three phases. How fast you progress is up to you. When the physical demands of a phase become routine and intuitively you feel you can move up to the next phase, give it a try. You might need a month in Phase 1, especially if you're reintroducing exercise after an extended time off. Even though the duration of the Phase 1 and Phase 2 cardio sessions is the same, thirty minutes, Phase 2 is more challenging because of the higher-intensity interval workouts. You might stay there longer, six weeks, for example. Phase 3, for long-term maintenance, devotes one session a week to an hour workout (more if you can handle it). These sustained efforts burn a lot of calories and train your metabolism to draw on fat stores for fuel. But variety is important here—you don't want to overtax the same muscles you've been training all week. So, for instance, if you jog your regular half-hour cardio sessions, the hour-long session might be a bike ride.

Reba uses a "perceived exertion scale," from 1 to 10, to measure the intensity with which you do the sessions. A relaxed steady lope might be a 5, a peppier effort might be a 7, and above 8, you're pushing into the anaerobic range—talking is difficult or impossible; breathing becomes deeper and faster and a bit labored. You'll only be able to sustain this for a minute or two at a time.

In Phase 2, every third session will be an interval workout. You'll alternate going hard for two minutes (perceived exertion in the 8 to 9 range), running or swimming or cycling or whatever you're doing, and then going easy for two minutes (perceived exertion below 5), for a total of thirty minutes. You'll burn a lot more calories at these higher intensities.

Cardio Program

Phase 1 / Building a Base

Activity: Walking, Swimming, Pool Aerobics, Paddling, Kayaking, Rowing, Elliptical, etc.

Duration: 30 minutes

Intensity: Any effort that you can maintain comfortably at a steady pace; perceived exertion 5 to 7 on a scale of 1 to 10

Frequency: Five to seven days per week

Phase 2 / Adding Intensity and Intervals

Activity: Walking, Swimming, Pool Aerobics, Paddling, Kayaking, Rowing, Elliptical, etc.

Duration: 30 minutes

Intensity: Every third day becomes interval training day: alternate 2 minutes hard, 2 minutes recovery; perceived exertion is 8 to 9, followed by recovery below 5.

Frequency: Five to seven days per week

Phase 3 / Increasing Duration

Activity: Walking, Swimming, Pool Aerobics, Paddling, Kayaking, Rowing, Elliptical, etc.

Duration: 30 minutes, including the interval session every third day. But lengthen one noninterval session per week to 60+ minutes

Intensity: This longer session can begin at a perceived exertion of 6 and progress to 7

Frequency: Five to seven days per week

Sculpting the Body: Body Composition

Addressing strength work brings us to the subject of body composition. It's incredibly important! Women can pay so much attention to the number on the scale, they ignore their muscle tone, specifically how much fat and how much lean muscle their frames are carrying. (Dress or slacks size is a better indicator of body composition than weight, but it's far from perfect—witness the number of thin, unfit women, the TOFIs, "thin on the outside, fat on the inside.") Having an adequate amount of muscle offers protection against the metabolic ravages of aging, like type 2 diabetes and heart disease, as well as against falls in the senior years that too often result in a broken hip and a loss of independence. There is weight-loss payoff as well. Increasing our muscle mass will increase our resting metabolism; in other words, the amount of calories we burn just by being alive. "It's a small but significant effect," Reba says. "And we want to use every advantage we have."

So how much time you invest in strength training every week will, according to Reba's plan, depend on how much you need it. If you are low on muscle based on your body fat measurement, work up to three sessions per week of thirty to sixty minutes each. Check the list on the next page that breaks out four measurable aspects of body shape. The most common, body mass index or BMI, is probably the least useful because it doesn't make a distinction between muscle weight and fat weight. But if you don't fall within the recommended range for any of the other three measures—waist circumference, waist-hip ratio, or the body adiposity index (BAI)—then we're going to recommend three strength workouts a week, in addition to the five to seven cardio sessions. Otherwise, two strength sessions will do the trick.

Of these three body measures, the one you likely won't be familiar with is the body adiposity index. Emerging research suggests that for women, your BAI score may be a better predictor of heart health than other conventional body shape measurements. And no math required. Just go on the Web site listed in the table, plug in your gender, age, height and hip circumference, and receive your number. Or, if you prefer, go to the gym and get a trainer to measure skinfolds with a caliper. You should get a similarly useful result.

Body Mass Index (BMI)

What it measures and optimal target:

- Height and weight are used to calculate BMI.
- A BMI of 18–25 is considered to be in the healthy range.

What it means:

- Limited value since it does not take into account one's body composition (muscle, bone, water).
- Assess other markers along with BMI.

Waist Circumference* (inches)

What it measures and optimal target:

- Waist measurement of less than 35 inches (women).
- Waist measurement of less than 43 inches (men).

What it means:

- High waist measurements are associated with more abdominal and visceral fat (fat around organs) and health risks (diabetes, heart disease, cancer).

---

* To measure your waist circumference, use a tape measure. Start at the top of the hip bone, then bring it all the way around—level with your navel. Make sure it's not too tight and that it is parallel with the floor. Don't hold your breath while measuring.

Waist: Hip Ratio (W:H)

What it measures and optimal target:

- W:H range less than .8–.86 (women)
- W:H range less than 1.0 (men)

What it means:

- Another measure of health risks associated with excess abdominal and visceral fat.

Body Composition

What it measures and optimal target:

- Can be measured a number of different ways, including special scales, skinfold calipers, etc.
- Body adiposity index (BAI) is a newer estimate of body fat.

What it means:

- BAI is derived from a calculation that takes into account gender, age, height, and hip circumference.
- Calculate your BAI at: http://easycalculation.com/health/body-adiposity-index.php.
- A healthy range of body fat is gender and age specific; go to the link above and see the interpretation based on the research to date.

Healthy BAI Ranges

AGE	WOMEN	MEN
20–39	21–33%	8–21%
40–59	23–35%	11–23%
60–79	25–38%	13–25%

How you want to go about getting stronger is up to you. It might be anything from resistance bands or dumbbells and ankle weights that you can use at home to making use of the full complement of resistance training machines at a gym. To get results, and to avoid getting hurt, you need to know what you're doing. That means working with a trainer or a physical therapist at least for the first couple of sessions. And you need to make sure that you're working out the six major muscle groups: chest, upper back, shoulders, abdomen, lower back and lower body. (Pilates is a great toner for the core muscles in the abdomen and the lower back, but just because you may have a wonderful Pilates class, don't think that you can skip the other four muscle groups!)

As you'll see in Reba's list below, you move through three phases. Progress is individual but a reasonable benchmark might be:

- Four to six weeks in Phase 1
- Four to six weeks in Phase 2
- Phase 3 for long-term maintenance

The frequency stays the same—two or three sessions per week, which should take no more than thirty minutes per session—but, no surprise, the challenge increases. In Phase 2, for example, you'll do fewer repetitions at higher intensity (stiffer resistance) before hitting the fatigue wall, when you no longer have enough strength to do another repetition with proper form. (What constitutes proper form depends on the exercise. Follow your trainer's lead.) In Phase 3, you'll stay at this higher intensity—it's a more efficient way to build muscle—but you'll be doing two sets of exercises for each muscle group, not one.

Strength Training Regimen

Phase 1

Duration: Suggested four to six weeks

Type: Six major muscle groups

Mode: Any (handheld weights, machines, water weights, body weight, resistance bands, etc.)

Frequency: Two to three times per week, depending on body fat measurement

Sets: One per area

Intensity: 10 to 15 reps to fatigue

Phase 2

Duration: Suggested four to six weeks

Type: Six major muscle groups

Mode: Any (handheld weights, machines, water weights, body weight, resistance bands, etc.)

Frequency: Two to three times per week, depending on body fat measurement

Sets: One per area

Intensity: Increase resistance; 8 to 12 reps to fatigue

Phase 3

Duration: Maintenance

Type: Six major muscle groups

Mode: Any (handheld weights, machines, water weights, body weight, resistance bands, etc.)

Frequency: Two to three times per week, depending on body fat measurement

Sets: Two per area

Intensity: 8 to 12 reps to fatigue

Flexibility and Balance

At the end of a full session, thirty minutes of cardio, twenty to thirty minutes of strength work, finish out with five to ten minutes of stretching. The muscles will be warmed up and more malleable then. A physical therapist can help you recognize tight muscles that will benefit from stretching and work with you on a personalized stretching routine that hits the key muscles. The usual drill: holding a stretch for twenty to thirty seconds in a static position to lengthen the soft tissues.

In a weight-loss-oriented program, you may not need special work on balance unless you're training to get better at a particular sport. Take this test: stand on one leg and bring the other leg up so that the thigh is parallel to the floor. If you can hold that position for thirty seconds without holding on to anything and without much wobble, you pass—balance exercises don't need to be a priority now. (But make sure to test both legs.) If you can't balance for thirty seconds, then incorporate five to ten minutes of these leg lifts into your workout until your balance improves.

Work Spa

Making time for exercise is an issue for most of us. One tip: you can subtract minutes from your dedicated workouts by putting in some minutes at the office. Stair walking is a great cardio workout for the high-rise-office set. And here are two resistance exercises that can be done in an office setting without attracting *too* much attention to yourself. Besides building up strength and flexibility, you're relieving stress and breaking up the amount of time you spend motionless in your chair—some researchers consider prolonged sitting to be a health risk factor on par with smoking!

1. Core/lower-body exercise: Stand, holding the back of a stable chair for balance. Sink into a squat position, pushing hips far back and lowering until thighs are parallel to the floor. Use core and legs to stand, lifting the chest. Or you can invest in a stability ball. Sitting and balancing on it, you're working your core and leg muscles continuously without even thinking about it.

If a large inflatable ball would attract too many stares in the office, use it at the beginning or the end of the workday or during the lunch hour.

2. Back/posture exercise: While either sitting or standing, grab a resistance band at either end and place it in front of you, across your body at chest level, your elbows bent at ninety degrees. At the start, your hands should be slightly wider than shoulder width apart. Then tighten the abdominal muscles and stretch the band by bringing your shoulder blades together. Hold for ten seconds. Slowly return to the original position and relax for ten seconds. Repeat ten times.

DANCING AND SHAKING

Here's a stress-busting and energy-lifting practice dreamed up, and intensively researched, by Dr. James Gordon, the founder and director of the Center for Mind-Body Medicine (cmbm.org) in Washington, DC. First, put on some fast-tempo music for seven to ten minutes. Close your eyes, plant your feet comfortably apart, let your arms hang loose by your sides, let your knees bend, keep breathing regularly and shake or bounce to the music. When the music is over, stop and feel the energy in your body that you've stirred up. Then put on a favorite song and dance to it however your body feels like moving.

Mind-Body-Spirit

Marian

I work with a lot of busy doctors like Marian, who has a thriving family-medicine practice in the Berkshires that doesn't leave her much time to take care of herself. I'd been seeing Marian for a few weeks for that stubborn ten-pound weight issue along with an assortment of digestive symptoms, and we weren't seeing much change. Then we decided to tackle her stress issues head-on. I got her to agree to do a simple belly-breathing exercise in between patient visits, when she was updating her records—she put a Post-it on her computer screen to remind herself. Then I encouraged her to take a good look at her office, where she spent so many hours during the day. Did it reflect a healing environment? She added some plants and a bowl of fresh fruit on her desk. And we found a yoga class in the area that she tries to get to twice a week, most weeks. It's enough to get her to begin to catch her breath, to appreciate her work as a healer for her patients and how important it is to take care of herself. These simple changes led to some other healthier choices, and two months in, Marian had lost five of the ten pounds that were bothering her and her irritable bowel symptoms had markedly improved. As it turned out, her eating habits weren't the main issue. It was the rest of her life.

I've been using a techniques like affirmation and visualizations with my nutrition clients for most of my career. But when I came to Kripalu seven years ago, I witnessed the power of mind-body practices such as yoga and qigong to support both weight loss and digestive health. Those of us with weight and gut issues have in some real sense lost touch with our bodies, how they want to look and feel. By focusing our attention on the physical self in a positive way, how we can bend and reach and stretch, even just a few basic techniques can wake us up! Although yoga hails from India and qigong from China, both traditions conceptualize their mission in a strikingly similar way. They are concerned with accessing and intensifying the life energy that courses through us—*prana* in Sanskrit, *qi* in Chinese. You could say that the Swift Diet is devoted to strengthening and nourishing the "digestive and metabolic *qi*"!

Whether you believe in the physical reality of this life energy or not, research strongly suggests that the attention we bring to these mind-body techniques can carry over from the mat to the everyday decisions we make about selecting, preparing and eating our meals. In one of my favorite studies, University of Washington epidemiologist Alan Kristal analyzed data on some fifteen thousand people. Those who had been overweight in their forties but who had taken up yoga for at least four years lost, on average, five pounds in their fifties. Remember, the vast majority of these people were not following a formal weight-loss program. And their counterparts, the ones who had not taken up yoga, gained, on average, eighteen and a half pounds!

An Australian study went the opposite methodological route and studied the intimate thoughts of a small group of overweight women taking a three-month yoga course. In their diaries, the women reported that as they began to feel more connected to their bodies, their eating habits improved: they made healthier food choices, ate less and ate more slowly. And in one small study by an Indian research group, yoga was found to be more effective than conventional drug therapy in treating IBS symptoms.

While the traditional yoga literature speaks to yoga's health benefits, no less a modern medical authority than Dr. Chutkan, herself a practitioner of yoga, talks about its ability to help relieve uncomfortable symptoms like bloating and gas and to build up the core abdominal muscles that support good gut health. At Kripalu, senior yoga teacher Vandita Kate Marchesiello and I are teaming up to teach simple yoga practices that promote digestive resiliency and increased flexibility, stamina and strength in the muscles and joints.

I've enlisted the help of two dear friends to introduce you to some basic yoga and qigong techniques specifically designed to support digestion and weight loss. My qigong teacher, Dr. Yang Yang, who earned a kinesiology PhD at the University of Illinois, teaches this venerable Chinese practice to cancer patients at Manhattan's prestigious Memorial Sloan Kettering Cancer Center and to students at his own Center for Taiji Studies, also in Manhattan. Yoga instructor Jenne Young teaches yoga at Kripalu and at other studios in the Berkshires as well as to patients at Berkshire Health Systems. Together she and I have co-led nutrition-and-digestive-health-meets-yoga workshops all over the country, including at the famous Rancho La Puerta spa outside of San Diego.

By closing this chapter with techniques drawn from both yoga and qigong, I'm inviting you to try something on, almost like a piece of clothing. Shop this section until you find a few things that fit your life and that you can look forward to doing with joy.

Yoga 101

People are who aren't so familiar with yoga tend to think of it as a collection of stretching poses. But the tradition, going back to the second-century Indian sage Pantanjali, is much richer than that, encompassing philosophy, meditation, breathing exercise and yes, the poses or *asanas*. Fundamentally, yoga is about the union of mind, body and spirit. Jenne's work with our students delves into all of this in a multiday immersion. Here's a step-by-step introductory session. Experiment with it. Try it out every day for a week. Each posture should take five to ten minutes.

Equipment: a yoga mat and a cushion or folded blanket.

1. Sitting pose: We'll start in Sukhasana or "Easy Pose," a comfortable cross-legged position. Sit on the edge of a folded blanket or cushion to support the natural curvature of your spine. Bending your right knee, bring your right heel in toward your groin. Bring the left foot to rest on the floor in front of your right leg or tuck it beneath the right shin. If you find that your knees are above the hips, add another blanket to raise you up, or

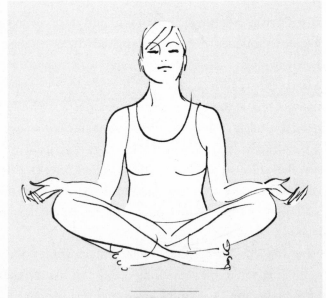

Sitting pose

support your knees with a cushion or rolled blanket. The idea is not to strain your knees but to allow them to relax. Root your sitting bones down as you lengthen out of the hips. Stack your shoulders over the hips and draw your shoulder blades back and down to open the chest. The crown of your head rises toward the ceiling. Gently tuck your chin to lengthen the back of your neck. Rest your hands on your thighs.

2. **Dirgha breath:** Still in the sitting position, we'll begin with a basic breathing exercise, the three-part yogic breath or, as it's called, Dirgha breath, which means "slow and deep." In this breath, we use the full capacity of our lungs, warming up the system, oxygenating the blood, getting rid of toxins and calming the body. We'll do ten Dirgha breaths. For each, slowly begin to inhale, filling the bottom of the lungs. Feel the belly expand. Continue inhaling and feel the middle section of the lungs under the rib cage expand so that the rib cage gently pushes up and out to the sides. Con-

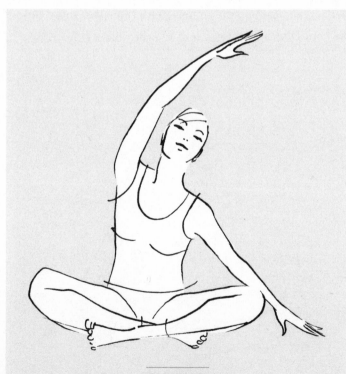

Side bends

tinue inhaling into the upper region of the chest, completely filling the lungs. Slowly exhale, letting go of the breath from the top of the lungs, then from the rib cage and finally exhaling all the air out of the belly. Squeeze the air out with your abdominal muscles, gently pulling the belly button back toward the spine.

3. Side bends: Now we're going to introduce movement, side bends, which are helpful for digestion because they stretch and strengthen the abdominal area and assist in relieving gas. After your last Dirgha breath, inhale and lengthen your torso, arms at your side. On the exhale, press your left hand on the mat. When you inhale, sweep your right arm up and arch it over to the left for a side bend. Keeping your sitting bones evenly grounded, take two full breaths, deepening into the side stretch. On the third inhale, come back to the center. Exhale and press your right hand on the mat. Inhale and sweep your left arm up and over to the right. Take two full breaths here, deepening into the side stretch on the right. On the third inhale, come back to the center. Repeat this two more times on each side. Take your time and enjoy.

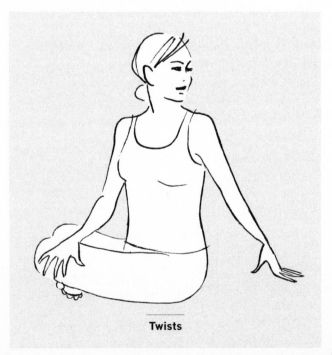

Twists

4. Twists: Back to the center and still in the sitting position, we move into twists. Twists can improve digestion by relieving tension in the torso. They massage and stimulate the entire abdominal area, helping to relieve constipation, gas and bloating. To begin, lengthen your arms out to the sides, take your right hand to your left knee and place your left hand behind you, pressing into the floor directly behind your tailbone. Inhale and lengthen the crown of your head toward the ceiling. Exhale and slowly begin to twist your torso to the left. Begin by twisting your belly first, then the rib cage, then the shoulders, gently turning your head to look over your left shoulder. The head is the last thing that turns. Stay in the twist for two full breaths. With each inhale think of lengthening the crown of your head toward the ceiling; with each exhale, deepen into the twist. On the third inhale, begin to slowly unwind back to the center. As you exhale, bring your hands back down by your side. Repeat the twist on the other side. Do a total of three twists on each side.

5. Cat and Cow: Slow movement between these two poses helps bring circulation to your abdominal organs. It also gently stretches the spine and helps relieve tension there that can disrupt good digestion. From the seated position, come into Table posture by bringing your hands directly under your shoulders. Your hips should be directly over your knees. You can place your blanket under your knees if they need extra support. Spread your fingers out wide and press into your fingers as well as your palms to create

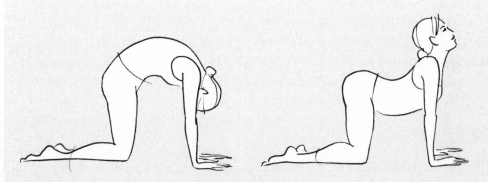

Cat and Cow

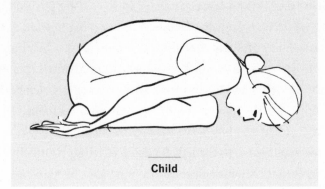

Child

a strong foundation. On the inhale, lift your shoulders and tailbone toward the ceiling while you gently press your belly toward the mat. You should be looking straight ahead. On the exhale, drop your tailbone and shoulders toward the mat and begin to round your spine toward the ceiling. Gently tuck your chin toward your chest. Repeat this cow and cat movement five more times. Cow is when the belly is pressing toward the floor; cat posture is when your spine is rounding toward the ceiling.

6. Child: Now, we move into the Child pose. This is a resting pose that gently stretches and stimulates the stomach and lower bowels to aid in digestion. It also relaxes the nervous system, essential to good digestion. Come into a neutral Table position and begin to draw your hips back toward your heels. Your belly comes to rest on your thighs; your arms can be out in front or back alongside your legs. Your forehead is resting on the floor or blanket. Relax into this folded posture. After three relaxing breaths, place your palms under your shoulders and push up into a Sukhasana comfortable seated position or whatever you like. Take a couple more cleansing breaths and savor a few minutes of quiet meditation.

Qigong 101

At Kripalu, I've had the good fortune to study qigong with many teachers, including Deborah Davis, Roger Jahnke, Robert Peng, Lee Holden and Dr. Yang Yang. Qigong means, literally, "energy work"—*qi* is the vital energy and *gong* is work. It's something of a catchall term that embraces a number of different Chinese traditions, from almost motionless meditations to the exquisitely athletic martial art of t'ai chi.

The career of Dr. Yang Yang is a good illustration of its scope. As a child growing up in China, he was diagnosed with a congenital heart defect. The family steered him to qigong training in hopes that it would improve his health, since expensive surgery during the Cultural Revolution was out of the question. The young Yang Yang outgrew his heart problem and grew into a t'ai chi champion. Now, as a qigong teacher in the States, he has returned to the therapeutic roots of the art, especially at Memorial Sloane Kettering Cancer Center, where he builds up the bodies and the spirits of cancer survivors.

I am a certified teacher in Dr. Yang Yang's school, but I have no ambition to master any difficult choreography. ("Empty movements," he calls it; that is, if the student hasn't developed the meditational foundation.) I, and many of my clients, have fallen in love with simple repetitive movements that are married to the rhythm of the breath. To the outsider, it may look very simple. But when you're doing it, you feel like you are drawing on and building up an energy, very real and powerful, that can be your ally in weight loss and digestive health.

As for the Western research, it's in its infancy, but promising. For instance, an Australian study examined whether regular qigong practice would have any physiological impact on a group of forty-one men and women with elevated blood sugar. After three months, the qigong group was found to have improved their blood sugar levels and lost more weight than a comparable group receiving standard medical care.

Here are three qigong exercises I've adapted from Dr. Yang Yang's program that will serve as an introduction. Try them for a week and see how you find them. The sequence shouldn't take more than fifteen minutes—it's both relaxing and energizing.

"Grand Opening and Closing" Slow Movement (five minutes): Assume a natural standing stance, feet even, slightly more than shoulder width apart, knees slightly bent. On the inhale, open the chest and extend the arms upward and outward in a circular motion, the palms facing out. Have the

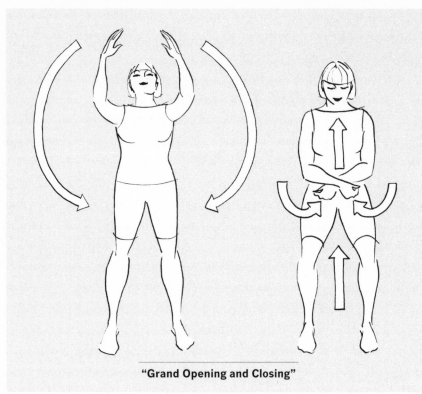

"Grand Opening and Closing"

intention of rising, of expanding. Feel free to gently shift your weight to one side. On the exhale, close the chest, drop your arms downward and cross them, continuing the circular motion and bending slightly and comfortably at the knee. Have the intention of sinking, of compacting, and move slowly, gracefully, as if you are in water. If you shifted your weight as you rose, then shift your weight to the other side as you contract and come down. Repeat this movement eight times for a total of nine times, and remember to smile!

Lying Down Qigong Meditation (five minutes): Lie down on a mat or a blanket. Make sure you are comfortable. You are giving the body time to find an optimal resting point. Empty the body! Put your hands on a spot two to three inches below the belly button, your "dantian" or "energy center," where the qi collects and is distributed throughout the body. Imagine you are stretched out on the beach and your body is slowly sinking into the sand, starting with the head. Picture the imprint of your head in the sand. Move down to the neck, which is sinking, then to your shoulders, then your middle back, lower back and pelvis, one area at a time. Then move down to the lower legs and finally to the feet. As your body is sinking in sequence, scan for any tension; if you notice any, just acknowledge it, breathe and relax. Use your imagination. Don't push; relax and sink. Close your eyes and ears and imagine your dantian. Have a gentle smile and beautiful day at the beach. If you fall asleep, that's OK too.

"Washing Organs" Slow Movement (five minutes): Assume a natural stance, feet even, slightly more than shoulder width apart. Begin with your arms gently resting at your sides. Breathe normally. Bring both arms out to the side and raise them up over your head, following the slow movement with your eyes, gathering the energy from the universe as you do this. Then, with your palms facing down, let your hands drop very slowly in

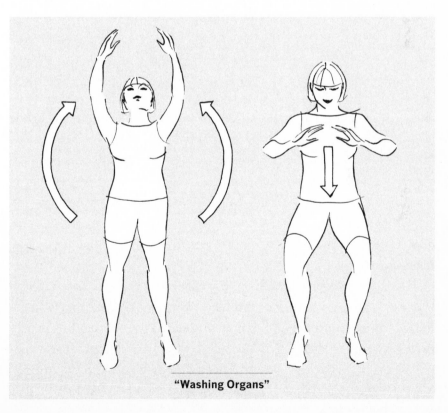

"Washing Organs"

front of you. Imagine that the energy you gathered from the universe fills each and every cell of your body as your hands float down in front of you, allowing the energy to flow through your body, organs, tissues and cells. Bend the knees slightly and comfortably as your arms come down. Breathe, relax and SMILE! Dr. Yang Yang says, "You are collecting energy from the universe and nature. It can be from the ocean, from the snow, from the mountain." Repeat this movement eight times for a total of nine times.

Swift Qi

So there you have it, the five elements of MENDS. If we've both done our jobs, you're inspired by the idea of bringing conscious intention into your life—into your food and meal choices, into your daily routines and into the mind-body practices that can rewardingly take us outside those routines. You've embraced a philosophy of "whole foods, whole person, whole life." You are suitably relaxed, open and ready to commit to the 4-week Swift Plan.

Chapter 7

THE 4-WEEK SWIFT PLAN

Week 1: Transition

It's time to get serious about creating a happy gut and a lighter, more resilient you. Beginning with this Transition week, we're removing the toxic foods that may be taxing your gut, and kick-starting recovery with their healthy counterparts. By the end of this week, you should be observing some physical changes. Which ones and at what pace will be different for everyone, but here are some typical experiences my clients have had after one week on the plan. The belly calms down: less gas and less bloat. The good bacteria in your belly are being fed properly and they're starting to work for, not against you. However, if your diet was very low in fiber before beginning the Swift Plan, you may experience a few days of increased gas and bloating before the belly begins to right itself. After a week off the added sugar, the cravings start to subside. You're no longer driving up your insulin levels and feeding the sugar craving at a metabolic level. You're not overstimulating those reward centers in the brain that lock in addiction at the neurological level.

Remove

- Sugar, gluten, dairy and the highest-FODMAP foods (see Finding High FODMAPs: The Swift List on p. 81)

- Processed foods with artificial sweeteners, colorings, preservatives and other toxic ingredients (see the Not-So-Swift Ingredients list on page 86)

Limit

- Grains (just a few servings of gluten-free grains this week)
- Alcohol (no more than two drinks per week)
- Caffeinated beverages (no more than one 8-ounce cup per day of coffee, or two cups of white, green or black tea)

Reflect: Set your intention for the week ahead. An intention is a positive statement in the present tense reflecting your goal. For example: "My digestive system is functioning well to support my healthy weight." "My food choices infuse my body with energy for a productive day."

Move: Begin the exercise plan in Chapter 6. Following the instructions there, take a body composition test to see whether you need two or three strength workouts per week to supplement your cardio workouts. If you're starting from scratch with exercise, here's a great first step: walk for ten minutes after at least two meals a day. It will improve digestion and begin to lay a fitness foundation.

Align: Experiment with either the yoga or qigong routines in Chapter 6; feel free to mix and match.

Food Prep: Take stock of your kitchen and remove the foods that no longer support your health, or your belly's. Review the menu plan and keep in mind that you're free to make substitutions. For example, if you're not a fan of tofu or are allergic to eggs, you can swap in a different breakfast option from another day. From there, create your shopping list and hit the stores. Take a look at my sample shopping list at the end of the next chapter.

Shop: Find the time that is convenient for you to shop. Shop smarter by following these simple guidelines:

1. Schedule shopping trips after you've had a meal; never shop when hungry.

2. Stick to your list so you're not distracted by nonessentials as you shop.

3. Know your local food shopping options to help get the highest food quality possible at a price that works with your budget.

Cook: One of the most essential ways to create a healthy belly is to do the majority of your own cooking, so you have to make time for it. Many of my clients find that taking a few hours over the weekend to cook for the week ahead works well, while others are happy to cook every night. The recipes that follow are a great introduction to home cooking, delicious but not fancy or time consuming. If you're not a recipe follower, check out my "do-your-own-thing" daily meal template in the FAQs section on p. 304. Whichever approach you prefer, keep these ideas in mind:

1. Wash and cut a selection of grab-and-go fresh veggies. Store in glass containers so your fridge "salad bar" is always ready to go for salads, stir-fries, soups or any other veggie-rich recipe from the menu. You have a green light for non-starchy vegetables (see the list on page 108) so feel free to add an extra serving of a cooked veggie side or a raw salad.

2. Make at least two of the dressings/marinades so they too are on hand for specific recipes or when you want to add a flavor boost to your meals.

3. Set yourself up to succeed by taking a couple of hours on your days off to do some "big batch" cooking. Make soups, prep proteins (marinate/ bake tofu and chicken for quick lunches and dinners), roast root vegetables, cook batches of steel-cut oats and quinoa. Freeze in individual portion-sized containers so there are lots of prepped, heat-and-eat options always within reach.

About snacks: I've included some snack ideas on page 285, but don't feel compelled to eat them. They're there if you're physically hungry. If a piece of fresh fruit suits you best, eat fruit, or mix it up with some of the other choices. This holds true for all four weeks of the Swift Plan.

Monday

Breakfast: Swift Smoothie: Berry Best (page 234)

Lunch: Spinach Salad with Basil Balsamic Salmon (page 250)

Dinner: Pecan-Crusted Chicken with Swiss Chard and Orange-Scented Carrots (page 263)

Tuesday

Breakfast: Carrot Ginger Power Cakes (page 223)

Lunch: Turkey Burger Vegetable Soup (page 251)

Dinner: Thai Vegetable Stir-Fry with Shrimp (page 274)

Wednesday

Breakfast: Get Up and Go Oats (page 227)

Lunch: Wrapped Fish with Veggies and Lemon Dill Dressing (page 253)

Dinner: Turkey Cutlets with Kiwi Salsa, Green Beans Almondine, In-Skin Baked Potato and Lemon Dill Dressing (page 275)

Thursday

Breakfast: Eggs Un-Benedict: Poached Eggs on Greens and Tomatoes (page 226)

Lunch: Chicken and Escarole Soup (page 240)

Dinner: Citrus Glazed Maple Salmon with Pineapple Cabbage Slaw (page 256)

Friday

Breakfast: Swift Smoothie: Kiwi Kraze (page 234)

Lunch: Asian Salad with Peanut Lime Tofu (page 237)

Dinner: Basil Balsamic Baked Chicken with Italian Herbed Zucchini (page 254)

Saturday

Breakfast: Thai Tofu Scramble (page 235)

Lunch: Kale Salad with Orange Zinger Chicken (page 244)

Dinner: Lemon Dill Shrimp with Sesame Bok Choy
(page 259)

Sunday

Breakfast: The Whites Stuffed: Classic Egg White and Veg Omelet
(page 236) with Green Ginger Veggie Juice (page 228)
Lunch: Quinoa Lentil Tabouli with Olive Herbed Pesto (page 246)
Dinner: Vietnamese Beef and Green Beans (page 278)

Take a moment: Place a drop of eucalyptus oil on your temple for an afternoon pick-me-up instead of your usual cup of coffee.

Week 2: Refinement

This second week, the Refinement phase, is about building on the successes of the first week. It's about getting comfortable with the idea of truly feeding the body, drawing strength from the phytonutrients, minerals and vitamins you're introducing into your system. Without processed foods and sugars to gum up the works, your gut, and the bacteria that live there, should move away from a state of imbalance, or dysbiosis, and toward a new resilience. By now, there's often marked improvement in those digestive problems. And a lot of my clients feel more energy at this stage. Because insulin levels have leveled out, more calories are being burned for energy, less stored as fat. At a deeper level, the large amount of antioxidants you're consuming is protecting your cells' power plant, the mitochondria, from damage.

Remove: Same as Week 1.

Limit: Same as Week 1.

Reflect: Think about your Transition week. Take note of the positive changes you've made as well as where you may have fallen a little short. Jot this down in your journal and use it as inspiration for the week ahead. Revisit your intention. Does it still resonate with you? Would you modify it for Week 2?

Move: Work on establishing a regular schedule and rhythm to both your cardio and strength workouts.

Align: By now, you've got some idea of what yoga and/or qigong movements suit you best. Begin to put together a brief daily routine, in the morning, to help launch your day, or in the evening, to help recover from it.

Food Prep: This week focuses on creative combinations and speedy meals with fewer recipes required. At the core of this week's refinements: plant-centric salads that work for lunch or dinner. If you've had a challenging day or just aren't feeling it in the kitchen, remember that you can always revisit any meal you particularly liked from Week 1. In this Refinement phase, you now have a few new meal ideas to work with, so cast a wider culinary net! And remember, dinner leftovers make great Swift and Simple lunches too, so feel free to make a little extra tonight and enjoy tomorrow.

Shop: This week is about expanding options, so check out the non-starchy vegetable list on page 108 in Chapter 4 to expand your veggie horizons. If spinach and kale were your go-to leafy greens, this week consider adding in arugula and watercress. Also add a fresh herb or two, such as parsley, cilantro or basil, in the salads. Capitalize on what's in season and on sale, and experiment! Add a never-tried-it-before vegetable such as jicama, kohlrabi, purple cauliflower or daikon radish to salads for extra texture and crunch. The idea is to push your culinary boundaries and expand the variety of nutrients on your plate.

Cook: Assembling the perfect lunch-in-a-bowl or packing it into a portable mason jar is a snap, particularly if you do the prep ahead of time. Chop and massage a bunch of lacinato (a.k.a. Tuscan or dinosaur) kale with a tablespoon of extra-virgin olive oil and 2 tablespoons of freshly squeezed citrus until it's well coated. Store in a glass container for a few hours or overnight. You now have the perfect foundation for a nutrient-dense lunch.

Layer 1: Leafy greens—at least 2 cups of arugula, spinach, romaine, watercress, mesclun greens, etc.

Layer 2: Crisp colorful veggies, 1 cup.

Layer 3: Herb (basil, dill, cilantro, parsley, etc.), ¼ cup.

Layer 4: Protein (canned fish, 2 hard-boiled eggs, cooked chicken, turkey, tofu, or lentils), 3 ounces.

Layer 5: Add-ons (olives, nuts, seeds), ¼ cup.

Layer 6: Dressing (any of the Swift dressings starting on page 280, or whisk up some extra-virgin olive oil, freshly squeezed lemon juice and herbs), 2 tablespoons.

For easy Swift Salads in a Jar: Use a mason jar (1 quart) to help with portability. Make sure you leave enough room at the top so when you're ready to eat, you can shake the jar to mix the ingredients. Using the food template below, assemble the layers so the dressing is on the bottom. Just before serving, give the jar a shake or two to distribute the dressing throughout the vegetables.

Layer 1: Dressing

Layer 2: Crisp vegetables that will withstand being in the dressing (carrots, cucumbers, radish, jicama)

Layer 3: Protein

Layer 4: Add-ons

Layer 5: Greens

Take a moment: Here's a pleasurable before-bed ritual borrowed from the traditional Indian health philosophy of Ayurveda. Before the lights go out, give yourself a five-minute foot massage with almond or coconut oil.

Week 3: Reintroduction

Congratulations! You've boosted your veggie intake. You're cooking more at home. You're doing your body, and your belly, proud! By this third week, you may notice less inflammation. It could be less muscle and joint pain; it could be a reduction in headaches. One area where many of my clients notice a difference is in their skin. Makes sense, doesn't it? Both the gut and the skin are the body's portals to the outside world, the inner skin and the outer skin, both colonized by a (hopefully) protective population of bacteria. A calmer gut and a body generally less buffeted by stress hormones means a more robust immune system in general, and often, a host of specific skin changes: dark circles under the eyes recede, acne clears up, psoriasis and eczema improve. The fastest skin changes usually occur when we eliminate foods and ingredients that are causing most of the problem, dairy and gluten being prime offenders.

If gut issues are still a major concern for you and you have not noticed a big improvement in your symptoms, consider staying with the Week 1 and 2 elimination diet for at least two more weeks. You can then reintroduce new foods more slowly, at your own pace. Follow the recipe for reintroduction that I lay out in detail at the end of this Week 3 section. If your digestion is in good shape, it's time to push out again and experiment with the reintroduction of cultured dairy products (for some, an introduction) and higher-FODMAP foods. If your now-more-resilient gut can handle them, they'll only enhance your weight loss and overall health. Enjoy the diverse range of recipes in the Week 3 meal plan, which includes legumes and fermented food, including cultured dairy products.

Introduce/Reintroduce

- Foods from the FODMAP "gang" (see Finding High FODMAPs: The Swift List on p. 81)
- Cultured dairy products and fermented foods

Continue

- To avoid sugar and gluten.
- To avoid processed foods such as artificial sweeteners, colorings, preservatives and other toxic ingredients (refer to page 86).
- Limiting alcohol (no more than two drinks per week).
- Limiting caffeinated beverages (no more than one 8-ounce cup of coffee a day or 2 cups white, green or black tea).

- To feel free to substitute any of your favorite recipes from the past two weeks if you have ones you'd like to repeat.

Move: Take stock of your cardio and strength program. If it's still challenging but doesn't leave you feeling washed out, stick with it. If you can go up in intensity, move up to a harder phase.

Align: If you have the time, hold the yoga poses longer or repeat the qigong moments more times, for a deeper, more meditative mind-body routine.

Reflect: Revisit your intention from Week 2. Again, does it need to be tweaked based on real-life experiences or pressures? Are there any concerns that have surfaced that need your attention? What would you like to achieve this week?

Food Prep: This week we take a Swift and Simple approach to making tasty smoothies that can be enjoyed for breakfast or as a snack if physical hunger strikes. With their perfect macronutrient balance of carbs, protein and fat, and minimal sugar content, these yogurt or kefir smoothies will help you find your fermented food comfort zone. (See the Swift Smoothie guide on page 233).

Shop: This week marks the return of dairy products to your shopping list, but not the conventional, factory-farmed, hormone- and antibiotic-treated kind. Your new go-to dairy will be organic, cultured yogurt and kefir, with small quantities of high-quality cheese if you like. You'll have a bit more to choose from in the produce section, as you'll be expanding your OK-to-experiment-with FODMAP foods to include items such as apples, mushrooms, garlic and onions. And you'll also welcome back some beans and legumes.

Cook: Get out your Crock-Pot and start slow-cooking hearty meals like Black Bean Sweet Potato Chili (page 239) and Slow Cooker Beef Stew (page 268). If you've been a bit slack on your day-off prep, no worries. One practice that works for some of my clients is the Veggie Prep Meditation, cleaning and chopping for the dinner meal ahead. In the morning or before bed, whichever you prefer, take ten minutes in the kitchen and assemble the veggies you'll be using for the next meal or two. Turn on some soothing instrumental music and start chopping. The idea is to focus on the task as a meditation rather than a dutiful means to an end. Notice the sounds, the smells, the beauty of what you're doing, and enjoy the peaceful activity. Be fully present in mind, body and spirit with your veggies!

About Snacks: Let go of the guilt if you find you have a physical hunger for a healthy snack! Use the snack list on page 285 to make a smart snack choice that nourishes your body and satisfies your taste buds.

Monday

Breakfast: Swift Smoothie: Creamsicle (page 234)
Lunch: Southwestern Salad with Avocado Cream Dressing
    (page 250)
Dinner: Orange Zinger Cod with Spinach and Cherry Tomatoes
    (page 261)

Tuesday

Breakfast: Eggs Un-Benedict: Poached Eggs on Greens and Tomatoes
    (page 226)
Lunch: Lauren's Lentil Soup (page 245)
Dinner: Turkey Sun-dried Tomato Meat Loaf with Roasted Red
    Rosemary Potatoes (page 276)

Wednesday

Breakfast: Sweet Potato Power Cakes (page 232)
Lunch: Hummus Veggie Wrap (page 243)
Dinner: Swift Nutty Fish with Lemon Asparagus (page 270)

Thursday

Breakfast: Chow Bella Chia Pudding (page 225)
Lunch: Black Bean Sweet Potato Chili (page 239)
Dinner: Slow Cooker Coconut Curry Chicken (page 269)

Friday

Breakfast: Basil and Egg Veggie Bake (page 230)
Lunch: Savory Salmon Cakes with Pink Sauerkraut
   (page 248)
Dinner: Taco Skillet Pie (page 271)

Saturday

Breakfast: Perfect Yogurt Parfait (page 231)
Lunch: Frittata Ratatouille with Arugula Salad
   (page 241)
Dinner: Slow Cooker Beef Stew (page 268)

Sunday

Breakfast: Thai Tofu Scramble (page 235)
Lunch: Unclassic Chicken Waldorf Salad (page 252)
Dinner: Moroccan Eggplant (page 260)

Take a moment: Skin brushing is an Ayurvedic method of pleasurably purifying the body. Buy a pair of raw silk gloves or a loofah sponge. Before bed or during downtime over the weekend, brush your entire body. Feel the friction bring a glow to the skin. Ayurvedic practitioners say that you are breaking up stagnation in the lymphatic system.

RECIPE FOR REINTRODUCTION

Starting Week 3, you've got a new job—dietary detective. You need to figure out if the foods that you're reintroducing into your diet are causing problems, in which case they need to go. You can try them again at a later date. There are a lot of different guidelines for reintroduction of foods, but here is the approach I use most often with clients. I described it briefly in Chapter 3, but here it is in more detail.

Directions

1. **Decide which food to reintroduce.** For example, if you suspect that apples might be bothering and bloating you, start by testing apples. Be sure to test only one food at a time.

2. **Track your experience.** Return to the diary you created back in Chapter 2 and create a record of your reactions to the test foods: safe to eat; unsafe with an adverse reaction; not sure, difficult to correlate symptoms with food ingestion. Remember, symptoms may go beyond the digestive ones. Adverse reactions can also cause fatigue, headache, brain fog, muscle aches and pain and skin rashes.

3. **Test for tolerance.** The test period lasts for three days, since you want to account for delayed food reactions, not just immediate and more obvious ones. You will consume a small amount of the test food in the morning on Day 1 and continue to increase the portion throughout the day, unless the first portion causes symptoms. For example, have half an apple at breakfast, the other half at lunch, and another apple later in the day. Do not eat any of the test food on Day 2 or Day 3 and continue to monitor and record your response if you have any.

4. **Reassess.** After the three-day test period, you are ready to move on and test other suspect foods (hopefully, there aren't many!). Follow the same reintroduction recipe as outlined.

5. **Remember the Rule of 3's:** If you are unsure a food caused your symptoms, test the food again at least three times on three separate occasions, three days apart.

Smoothies 101

In the Blender:

Protein: 1 cup plain, unsweetened organic yogurt or kefir.

Fruit (fresh or frozen): Berries, bananas, apples, oranges, mangos, pineapple, cantaloupe, avocados (1 cup).

Vegetables/Herbs: Greens: spinach, kale, chard, parsley, cilantro, dill, mint, watercress (1+ cup).

Add-ins (choose up to 3): 1 to 2 tablespoons nut butter, 1 to 2 teaspoons coconut (flakes, shredded), 1 teaspoon spices (ginger, cloves, cinnamon, nutmeg), 1 tablespoon flax/hemp/chia/pumpkin/sunflower seeds, 1 to 2 teaspoons cocoa powder/nibs, 1 to 3 pitted dates, ice if desired.

Liquid: ¼ cup water if using yogurt and no water if using kefir.

Seasoning with Herbs and Spices

My Personal Chef's Blend: Pick five herbs that appeal to you and make your own blend. Place in a small glass bottle to sprinkle on your food as desired. Or purchase ready-made herb and spice blends below.

Ready-made Herb and Spice Blends

- **Italian seasoning:** Marjoram, thyme, rosemary, savory, sage, basil, oregano and basil
- **Chinese five-spice:** Fennel, anise, ginger, licorice root, cinnamon and cloves
- **Curry powder:** Coriander, fenugreek, turmeric, cumin, black pepper, bay leaves, celery seed, nutmeg, cloves, onion, red pepper and ginger
- **Herbes de Provence:** Savory, marjoram, rosemary, thyme, oregano, fennel seeds and lavender
- **Garam masala:** Coriander, black pepper, cumin, cardamom and cinnamon
- **Poultry seasoning:** Thyme, sage, marjoram, rosemary, black pepper and nutmeg
- **Pumpkin pie spice:** Cinnamon, ginger, nutmeg and allspice

Note: McCormick, Frontier Seasonings, Simply Organic and Spice Hunter have organic spices and interesting spice blends.

Gas-busters!

Here are a few ways to cut the intestinal gas that some high-fiber foods can promote:

1. *Increase your bean consumption gradually.* You might start with ¼ cup per day and then slowly, over the course of one to two weeks, increase to 1 cup daily. You should find that your body adapts to this slow and steady progression.

2. *Soak beans overnight before cooking them.* This breaks down some of the gas-promoting oligosaccharides.

    a. To soak beans quickly, rinse and pick over the beans, cover them with water (1 part beans to 3 parts water) and boil the beans for 5 minutes. Let them sit for an hour and then cook thoroughly until softened.

    b. For a longer soak, rinse and pick over the beans, cover them in water (1 part beans to 3 parts water) and soak for 8 hours, or overnight. Drain and change the water before cooking thoroughly until softened.

    c. And, for slow cooking, your Crock-Pot is the perfect cooking vessel for beans. If time is of the essence, dust off your pressure cooker, a quick and easy cooking method that will deliver beans (and many other foods) cooked to perfection!

3. *Add some kombu strips to your beans.* Kombu is a sea vegetable that, according to macrobiotic tradition, may help increase the digestibility of beans. It certainly adds a boost of flavor!

4. *Toss in some carminatives.* Carminatives are herbs or herbal preparations that can decrease flatulence. In addition, these herbs can help facilitate digestion. Experiment with various herbs and herbal blends to find the most soothing combination:

    Anise

    Basil

    Caraway

    Cardamom

    Cinnamon

Coriander

Cumin

Dill

Fennel

Ginger

Marjoram

Mint (peppermint, spearmint, wintergreen)

Nutmeg

Oregano

Parsley

Rosemary

Sage

Savory

Thyme

My Carminative Tea or Broth: Make your own tea or broth by steeping your favorite herb(s). Savor a small cup at the end of a meal. You can also use it as a broth to add to dressings, marinades, sides or entrées.

My Carminative Choice: Chew on some fennel seeds, mint or sprigs of parsley for an après-meal digestive aid.

5. *Can it?* Canned beans are a time-saver. Just be sure to choose a brand such as Eden Foods that is not loaded with sodium, is free of BPA and, as an added benefit, contains kombu!

6. *Need an enzyme boost?* You can try Bean-zyme (vegetarian enzyme preparation) or Beano at the beginning of a legume meal. These products contain the enzyme alpha-galactosidase, which breaks down the sugar raffinose in the beans, cutting down on gas and possible digestive upset.

Week 4: Renewal

In this final, Renewal week you'll continue to internalize new habits and rituals to help mend your microbiota. Know that whatever tangible results you've enjoyed, success on the Swift Plan goes beyond a number on a scale.

You're returning the body to its vibrant state—the goal of renewal. By this fourth week, the mental changes may be as obvious as the physical ones. A month's worth of smart eating, good sleep, and attention to mind-body practices should translate to sharper, more focused mental functioning and a lighter, more buoyant feeling.

Continue

- To enjoy a bigger boost of prebiotic and fermented foods.
- To avoid sugar and gluten.
- To avoid processed food ingredients, such as artificial sweeteners, colorings, preservatives (see the list on page 86).
- Limiting alcohol (no more than two drinks per week).
- Limiting caffeinated beverages (no more than one cup of coffee a day or 2 cups white, green or black tea)
- Feel free to substitute any of your favorite recipes from the past three weeks if you have ones you'd like to repeat.

Reflect: Have you been integrating mindful practices? Eating more slowly? Detected any dairy distress or FODMAP feedback? Developed an interest in fermented foods? When going out with family or friends, do you find you're eating less? Are you more conscious of your alcohol intake?

Move: If you are doing thrice-weekly strength workouts, test your body composition again. If you pass, you can drop a weekly strength workout and concentrate more energy on calorie-burning cardio. Consider moving up a phase in the cardio workout to include either interval workouts or a slow, steady hour-long single workout.

Align: If yoga or qigong has become an important part of your day, explore what's available in your area in the way of regular classes. You'll likely find plenty of yoga options, from your local gym to a dedicated yoga studio. The qigong presence is growing nationally, including the more athletic, martial-arts-influenced version called t'ai chi.

Food Prep: This week is all about a Swift and Simple approach to creating satisfying vegan dinner bowls. The goal is to integrate the diverse plant foods from the past three weeks and spice them up with flavors from around the globe. You can substitute clean, lean animal protein, but I encourage you to stretch beyond your dietary comfort zone. Remember, just because it's dinner, it doesn't always have to include fish, meat, poultry or eggs.

Shop: Be on the lookout for colorful, seasonal veggies that will make up the bulk of your bowl. Think about color-coding and shop for at least four different produce colors. Allow your inner kitchen artist free play. The more colors in your bowl, the more nutrients in your body, so don't hold back.

Cook: Consider roasting a batch of vegetables over the weekend. Cook up ancient grains to be tossed in your bowl as a complement to the strong vegetable foundation. This is a great opportunity to review the produce in your fridge to check what's still fresh—and to salvage any items that may be about to pass their prime. And feel free to swap out any of the Swift meals. You can trade dinners for lunches, lunches for dinners, even breakfasts for dinners. The menu offerings are your palette—mix and match as much or as little as you like.

Bowl-Ology

Layer 1: Steamed/sautéed greens (kale, Swiss chard, collards, mustard, bok choy), at least 2 cups.

Layer 2: Crisp colorful veggies (roasted, steamed, sautéed or raw), at least 1 cup.

Layer 3: Protein (beans, lentils, tofu), 1 cup.

Layer 4: Fermented food (sauerkraut, tempeh, miso, pickles, kimchi, yogurt), to taste.

Layer 5: Ancient grains (amaranth, buckwheat, millet, quinoa, brown rice), bean noodles, ½ cup cooked.

Layer 6: Herb/spices (basil, dill, cilantro, parsley, etc.), to taste—refer to the "Ready-made Herb and Spice Blends" on page 217, to taste.

Layer 7: Add-ons (olives, nuts, seeds, avocados, sea vegetables), 1 to 2 tablespoons

Layer 8: Dressing/condiments: salsa, Swift dressings/marinades (page 280), hot sauce, tamari, olive oil, lemon, vinegar), 1 to 2 tablespoons

Take a moment: Find a quiet time to think about your occasional lapses on this healthy weight path. Accept that such lapses are inevitable. Forgive yourself and recommit to staying on your program. Remember the Intention Card you wrote in Chapter 2. Write a new one and place it in your purse or wallet for future use. Maybe it's identical to the original; maybe you've learned something new about your motivation for getting leaner and healthier. Incorporate that into the new card.

Chapter 8

RECIPES

The Swift Diet Menu Plan: Breakfasts

It's not morning without breakfast, or at least, it shouldn't be. Whether you like to eat your breakfast at the kitchen table, grab and go or have a civilized sit-down while reading the news, these breakfasts offer you a range of delicious day-starting options—which can also fill in as a post-workout snack or a light dinner when time is tight.

Try to avoid eating the same breakfast two days in a row, so that you continue to keep your taste buds and gut bacteria guessing.

Carrot Ginger Power Cakes

Prep Time: 10 minutes
Cook Time: 22 to 25 minutes
Makes: 12 muffins
Serves: 6 (2 muffins per serving)

INGREDIENTS

½ cup coconut flour
2 teaspoons ground cinnamon

½ teaspoon baking powder

2 teaspoons ground ginger

¾ cup carrot puree or organic carrot baby food

¼ cup walnut oil

6 large eggs

2 teaspoons pure vanilla extract

¼ cup 100 percent pure maple syrup

DIRECTIONS

Step 1. Preheat the oven to 350°F. Place 12 2½-inch unbleached paper muffin liners in a muffin tin.

Step 2. In a small mixing bowl, sift the coconut flour, cinnamon, baking powder and ginger together.

Step 3. In a large mixing bowl, whisk the carrot puree, walnut oil, eggs, vanilla and maple syrup until well blended.

Step 4. Add the sifted flour mixture to the carrot puree mixture and blend together until smooth.

Step 5. Divide the batter among the lined muffin cups.

Step 6. Bake for 22 to 25 minutes, or until a knife inserted in the middle of a muffin comes out clean. Let cool before serving.

Swift Tip

- Save baking time by doubling the recipe and freezing extra muffins for future use. Freeze muffins in individual containers for the ultimate, portion-controlled, grab-and-go breakfast. Drop a couple in your bag and after about 15 minutes of defrosting, the muffins are ready to eat.

Chow Bella Chia Pudding

Prep Time: 5 minutes plus 3 hours (chill time)
Cook Time: None
Serves: 2

INGREDIENTS

1 cup plain, unsweetened kefir or nondairy kefir such as coconut, almond, etc.

¼ cup chia seeds

2 teaspoons 100 percent pure maple syrup

Spice or pure flavor extract per Swift Twist variations (see below)

TOPPINGS

1 cup fresh seasonal fruit

2 tablespoons nuts, chopped

DIRECTIONS

Step 1. In a 1-quart sealable glass jar, add the kefir, chia seeds and maple syrup and shake until evenly mixed.

Step 2. Add the flavor boosters for desired variation below, seal the glass jar and shake again.

Step 3. Place the jar in the refrigerator and chill for at least 3 hours.

Step 4. Serve topped with fresh seasonal fruit (½ cup per serving) and chopped nuts (1 tablespoon per serving).

SWIFT TWISTS

Vanilla Almond: Add ½ teaspoon of pure vanilla extract at Step 2. Serve topped with fresh or frozen wild blueberries and chopped or slivered almonds.

Cocoa Cinnamon: Add ½ teaspoon ground cinnamon and ½ teaspoon unsweetened cocoa powder at Step 2. Serve topped with chopped walnuts and banana slices.

Banana Ginger: Add ½ teaspoon ground ginger and 1 small mashed banana at Step 2. Serve topped with chopped macadamia nuts.

Maple Walnut: Add ½ teaspoon maple extract at Step 2. Top with chopped walnuts.

Peanut Butter Chocolate: Add ½ teaspoon unsweetened cocoa powder and 1 tablespoon natural peanut butter at Step 2. Serve topped with banana slices.

Swift Tip

- Make a little extra to have on hand to stash in the office fridge so you'll reach for it as a healthy snack instead of a candy bar when hunger strikes.

Eggs Un-Benedict: Poached Eggs on Greens and Tomatoes

Prep Time: 5 minutes
Cook Time: 5 minutes
Serves: 1

INGREDIENTS

1 teaspoon raw apple cider vinegar

1 teaspoon extra-virgin olive oil

1 medium tomato, chopped

3 cups fresh baby spinach

2 large eggs

Sea salt and freshly ground black pepper to taste

1 cup fresh seasonal fruit

DIRECTIONS

Step 1. Fill a small pot about halfway with warm water and add the vinegar. Bring to a high simmer over medium-high heat.

Step 2. Meanwhile, in a small skillet over medium heat, add the olive oil, tomato and spinach and sauté for 3 minutes, stirring frequently.

Step 3. When the water comes to a high simmer, crack the eggs into the pot and cook for about 3 minutes, or until the whites are firm. Remove from the water with a slotted spoon and place over the tomato and spinach mixture. Season with salt and pepper to taste.

Step 4. Serve with fresh seasonal fruit.

Swift Tips

- Go beyond spinach and vary your greens—these eggs are also delicious on chard, kale, arugula, escarole, etc.
- To make this breakfast even more filling, sprinkle a teaspoon or two of chia seeds or ground flax over the veggies and dig in.

Get Up and Go Oats

Prep Time: 5 minutes
Cook Time: 20 to 25 minutes
Serves: 4

INGREDIENTS

3 cups water
1 cup steel-cut oats, certified gluten-free (rinsed and soaked overnight if desired)
1 teaspoon ground cinnamon
1 medium banana, sliced

4 tablespoons shelled walnuts

1 tablespoon unsweetened coconut flakes

DIRECTIONS

Step 1. In a medium pot, bring the water to a boil, add the oats, lower the heat to a simmer, add the cinnamon and cook for 20 to 25 minutes, until the oats are soft.

Step 2. Top with the banana, walnuts and coconut flakes.

Green Ginger Veggie Juice

Prep Time: 5 minutes

Cook Time: None

Serves: 1

INGREDIENTS

1 medium tomato

1 cucumber

1 carrot

1 cup greens

1 teaspoon ground turmeric

1 tablespoon grated fresh ginger (unpeeled if organic)

1 tablespoon freshly squeezed lime juice

½ cup water

DIRECTIONS

Step 1. Place all of the ingredients in a juicer or high-speed blender and process until smooth.

Swift Tips

- Let's get juiced! But let's do it right. Ideally, when you're making a healthy juice, go heavy on veggies and light on fruit. Fruit should add a touch of sweetness to your juice, not drown it with extra sugar. Think of fruit as the cherry on top—not the main event.
- If you have any leftovers, freeze in ice cube trays, then toss into soups, stews or marinara sauce for a phytonutrient boost.

Lox and Rolls: Simple Fish Roll-ups

Prep Time: 5 minutes
Cook Time: None
Serves: 1

INGREDIENTS

3 ounces wild-caught lox, nitrate-free and naturally smoked

1 cucumber, thinly sliced

1 tomato, thinly sliced

2 red radishes, thinly sliced

1 teaspoon horseradish (optional)

2 large Boston or green leaf lettuce leaves, washed and patted dry

2 tablespoons Lemon Dill Dressing (page 282)

DIRECTIONS

Step 1. Divide the lox, cucumber, tomato, radishes and horseradish on the lettuce leaves and drizzle with the dressing.

Swift Tips

- Look for a smoked wild salmon—my favorite brand is Ducktrap River of Maine.

- Lox will last 3 to 5 days in the fridge and longer if it's in the freezer and well wrapped.

Basil and Veggie Egg Bake

Prep Time: 10 minutes
Cook Time: 20 minutes
Makes: 12 muffins
Serves: 4 (3 muffins per serving)

INGREDIENTS

¼ cup diced bell peppers
¼ cup diced zucchini
1 cup frozen spinach, thawed and well drained
2 tablespoons feta cheese
6 large eggs
4 large egg whites
1 tablespoon chopped fresh basil or 1 teaspoon dried basil
1 tablespoon Parmesan cheese

DIRECTIONS

Step 1. Heat oven to 350°F. Use 12 2½-inch unbleached muffin liners. Distribute the bell pepper, zucchini, spinach and feta cheese equally in the lined muffin cups, covering the bottom.

Step 2. In a large mixing bowl, whisk together the eggs, egg whites, basil and Parmesan cheese and then pour the egg mixture over the veggies until each muffin cup is half to three-quarters full.

Step 3. Bake for 20 minutes, or until a knife inserted in the middle of a muffin comes out clean.

Swift Tips

- Stash a few in the freezer at the office and warm one up in the toaster oven before you head out for your post-work Zumba class. It will give you the energy you need to fuel your workout and keep you from being ravenous afterward.
- If you're headed to a cocktail party, snack on a muffin beforehand so you don't overdo it on hors d'oeuvres.

Perfect Yogurt Parfait

Prep Time: 2 minutes
Cook Time: None
Serves: 1

INGREDIENTS

1 cup plain, unsweetened organic yogurt

¼ teaspoon spice (ground cinnamon, ground ginger, ground nutmeg, etc.) or ½ teaspoon pure flavor extract (vanilla, maple, orange, etc.)

1 cup fresh or frozen berries

1 tablespoon chopped nuts

1 tablespoon seeds (sunflower, pumpkin, flax or chia)

DIRECTIONS

Step 1. In a glass or single-serving bowl, mix the yogurt with the spice or pure flavor extract.

Step 2. Serve topped with fruit, nuts and seeds.

Swift Tip

- You'll never get bored with the Perfect Parfait—the possibilities are endless. Try healthy add-ins like cinnamon, ginger and nutmeg and experiment with different fruits to keep your taste buds interested!

Sweet Potato Power Cakes

Prep Time: 10 minutes
Cook Time: 22 to 25 minutes
Makes: 12 muffins
Serves: 6 (2 muffins per serving)

INGREDIENTS

½ cup coconut flour

2 teaspoons ground cinnamon

½ teaspoon baking powder

2 teaspoons ground nutmeg

¾ cup sweet potato puree or organic sweet potato baby food

¼ cup walnut oil

6 large eggs

2 teaspoons pure vanilla extract

¼ cup 100 percent pure maple syrup

DIRECTIONS

Step 1. Preheat the oven to 350°F. Place 12 2½-inch unbleached paper muffin liners in a muffin tin.

Step 2. In a small mixing bowl, sift the coconut flour, cinnamon, baking powder and nutmeg together.

Step 3. In a large mixing bowl, whisk the sweet potato puree, walnut oil, eggs, vanilla and maple syrup until well blended.

Step 4. Add the sifted flour mixture to the sweet potato puree mixture and blend together until smooth.

Step 5. Divide the batter among the lined muffin cups.

Step 6. Bake for 22 to 25 minutes, or until a knife inserted in the middle of a muffin comes out clean. Let cool before serving.

Swift Smoothie

Prep Time: 5 minutes
Cook Time: None
Serves: 1

INGREDIENTS

8 to 12 ounces cold water (use more water if you like it thinner)
Fruit: ½ small banana (peeled and then frozen)
½ cup fruit, frozen or fresh in season
Vegetable: 1 cup fresh or ½ cup frozen green of your choice (spinach, kale, watercress, etc.)
Protein: 2 level tablespoons raw, unsalted nut or seed butter
Spice: A dash of spice of your choice (ground ginger, ground nutmeg, ground cinnamon, orange peel, etc.)
Optional: You can add a protein powder if you would like an even higher protein boost; one of my favorites is Omega Nutrition pumpkin seed protein powder.

DIRECTIONS

Step 1. Place all of the ingredients in a blender and blend on medium speed until smooth (20 to 30 seconds).

SWIFT TWISTS

You can adapt the basic recipe in a variety of ways, but here are a few more of my favorites:

Berry Best: ½ banana; ½ cup blueberries; 1 cup leafy greens; 2 tablespoons raw, unsalted almond butter; 8 to12 ounces cold water

Creamsicle: ½ banana; 1 orange, seeded and peeled; 1 cup leafy greens; ½ tablespoon coconut butter; 2 tablespoons macadamia nut butter; 8 to 12 ounces cold water

Kiwi Kraze: ½ banana; 1 peeled kiwi; 1 cup leafy greens; 2 tablespoons raw, unsalted almond butter; 8 to 12 ounces cold water

Tropical Treat: ½ banana, ½ cup pineapple, 1 cup leafy greens, ½ tablespoon coconut butter, 2 tablespoons macadamia nut butter, 8 to 12 ounces cold water

Peanut Butter Chocolate: 1 banana, 1 cup spinach, 2 tablespoons peanut butter, ½ teaspoon unsweetened cocoa powder, ½ teaspoon ground cinnamon, 8 to 12 ounces cold water

Strawberry Dream: ½ banana; 1 cup frozen unsweetened strawberries; 1 cup leafy greens; 2 tablespoons raw, unsalted almond butter; 8 to 12 ounces cold water

Swift Tips

- No time in the morning to assemble smoothie ingredients? Before you go to bed, combine all of the ingredients except the water in the blender cup and store overnight in the fridge. In the morning, simply add the liquid and hit the blend button.
- If you've made a bit too much or have a little leftover smoothie, don't toss it. Instead, pour the excess into ice cube trays, freeze, and toss the frozen smoothie cubes into your next smoothie.

Thai Tofu Scramble

Prep Time: 10 minutes

Cook Time: 13 minutes

Serves: 4

INGREDIENTS

1 tablespoon extra-virgin coconut oil

½ cup diced bell peppers

½ cup grated carrots

¼ cup chopped scallions (green part only)

½ cup coconut milk (see Swift and Simple Additive-free Homemade Coconut Milk, page 236)

2 teaspoons green curry paste

1 teaspoon ground turmeric

1 tablespoon gluten-free tamari

1 pound firm tofu, rinsed, drained and crumbled

2 cups chopped fresh spinach or 1 cup frozen spinach, thawed and well drained

DIRECTIONS

Step 1. In a large sauté pan over medium heat, add coconut oil, bell peppers, carrots and scallions and sauté for 3 minutes.

Step 2. Add the coconut milk, green curry paste, turmeric and tamari and stir until dissolved.

Step 3. Stir in the crumbled tofu and simmer for about 8 minutes.

Step 4. Add the spinach and cook for another 2 minutes.

Swift Tips

- Unlike eggs, you can reheat tofu without radically changing the texture, so don't be afraid to make a little extra and save a batch for another meal.
- Swift and Simple Additive-free Homemade Coconut Milk: Add 1 tablespoon creamed coconut (brand: Let's Do . . . Organic Creamed Coconut) to 8 ounces hot water in a blender and process until smooth. Transfer to a glass jar and store in the refrigerator for up to 5 days.

The Whites Stuffed: Classic Egg White and Veg Omelet

Prep Time: 5 minutes

Cook Time: 10 minutes

Serves: 1

INGREDIENTS

2 teaspoons extra-virgin olive oil

3 tablespoons diced tricolored peppers

1 tablespoon chopped fresh tomato

1 tablespoon chopped fresh parsley

½ cup chopped fresh spinach

3 large egg whites

Pinch of sea salt and freshly ground black pepper (optional)

DIRECTIONS

Step 1. In a small skillet over medium heat, add the olive oil and peppers and sauté until soft.

Step 2. Stir in the tomato and cook for 1 to 2 minutes.

Step 3. Add the parsley and spinach and cook until wilted.

Step 4. Mix in the egg whites, folding over the omelet, allowing the eggs to cook until desired consistency.

Swift Tip

- Frozen peppers and spinach work almost as well as fresh. Just remember to thaw them the night before, store in the fridge until you're ready to cook, and squeeze out the extra moisture.

The Swift Diet Menu Plan: Lunches

Are you often "too busy" to eat lunch? For a lot of people, what they're really saying is they're at a loss to figure out what they should eat, especially when they don't have time to leave the office in search of a healthy lunch. On the Swift Plan, you won't have that problem because you'll be preparing your meals in advance, guaranteeing that every lunch is there when you need it, full of nutrients to power you through your day. And it will taste far more delicious than the same old sandwich from the corner deli!

Asian Salad with Peanut Lime Tofu

Prep Time: 10 minutes
Cook Time: None
Serves: 2

INGREDIENTS

4 cups shredded bok choy or green cabbage
1 cup fresh bean sprouts
1 red bell pepper, thinly sliced
½ cup sliced water chestnuts
¼ cup chopped fresh cilantro

Who Knew Tofu (see below)

4 tablespoons Peanut Lime Dressing (page 283)

DIRECTIONS

Step 1. Place the bok choy, bean sprouts, bell pepper, water chestnuts and cilantro in a bowl. Top with Who Knew Tofu and drizzle with the dressing.

Who Knew Tofu

(Made Ahead of Time)

Prep Time: 1 hour and 10 minutes

Cook Time: 25 to 30 minutes

Serves: 4

INGREDIENTS

1 pound firm tofu

MARINADE

2 tablespoons toasted sesame oil

2 tablespoons brown rice vinegar

1 tablespoon gluten-free tamari

1 teaspoon ground ginger

¼ cup water

"UN-BREADING"

1 teaspoon Chinese five-spice

¼ cup almond flour

DIRECTIONS

Step 1. Rinse and drain the tofu by gently pressing it with a linen cloth until the water comes out, then pat dry. Slice into eight pieces and place in a shallow baking dish.

Step 2. Combine the marinade ingredients in a glass measuring container and pour over the tofu. Marinate for at least 1 hour.

Step 3. Preheat oven to 375°F.

Step 4. In a medium bowl, add the Chinese five-spice seasoning to the almond flour. Remove the tofu from the marinade one piece at a time and dredge in the breading mixture. Coat both sides and place on an oiled baking sheet.

Step 5. Bake the tofu for 25 to 30 minutes, flipping it halfway through the baking time.

Black Bean Sweet Potato Chili

Prep Time: 20 minutes
Crock-Pot Time: 4 to 5 hours
Serves: 4

INGREDIENTS

1 medium red onion, chopped

1 green bell pepper, chopped

3 cloves garlic, minced

1 tablespoon chili powder

1 tablespoon ground cumin

¼ teaspoon ground cinnamon

1 tablespoon unsweetened cocoa powder

1 28-ounce can fire-roasted diced tomatoes

2 15½-ounce cans black beans

1 large sweet potato (about 8 ounces), cut into ½-inch cubes

1 cup water

DIRECTIONS

Step 1. In a 4- to 6-quart slow cooker, combine the onion, bell pepper, garlic, chili powder, cumin, cinnamon and cocoa powder.

Step 2. Add the tomatoes, beans (and their liquid), sweet potato and water.

Step 3. Cover and cook until the chili has thickened and the sweet potatoes are tender (over high heat for 4 to 5 hours; over low heat for 7 to 8 hours).

Note: This recipe can also be made on the stovetop.

Chicken and Escarole Soup

Prep Time: 15 minutes

Cook Time: 1 hour and 30 minutes

Serves: 10 (1½ cups per serving)

INGREDIENTS

1 whole organic chicken (3 to 4 pounds)

10 cups water

2 tablespoons apple cider vinegar

1 fennel bulb, diced

3 carrots, diced

1 parsnip, diced

1 cup diced red bell pepper

1 bunch escarole, washed, trimmed and chopped

1 large sweet potato (about 8 ounces), diced into ½-inch cubes

2 tablespoons finely chopped fresh tarragon or 1 tablespoon dried tarragon leaves

2 tablespoons finely chopped fresh dill or 1 tablespoon dried dill

¼ teaspoon freshly ground black pepper

½ teaspoon sea salt

DIRECTIONS

Step 1. Clean the chicken inside and out.

Step 2. In a large stockpot, place the water, chicken and vinegar. Bring to a boil over high heat, then reduce the heat to medium-low and simmer uncovered for 30 to 40 minutes, until the meat starts to fall off the bone. Remove the chicken from the pot and let cool.

Step 3. Add the fennel, carrots, parsnip, bell pepper, escarole, sweet potato, tarragon, dill, pepper and salt to the pot and continue to simmer over medium-low heat for about 20 minutes, until vegetables are al dente.

Step 4. After the chicken is cool to the touch, debone, cut into chunks, and return to the pot. Simmer for about 30 minutes more or until the vegetables soften.

Frittata Ratatouille with Arugula Salad

Prep Time: 10 minutes

Cook Time: 35 to 40 minutes

Serves: 6

INGREDIENTS

1 medium red or purple potato (3 ounces), cut into ½-inch cubes

6 large eggs

5 large egg whites

1 teaspoon dried oregano

¼ teaspoon freshly ground black pepper

2 tablespoons grated Parmesan cheese

2 tablespoons feta cheese

1 tablespoon extra-virgin olive oil

1 shallot, chopped

1 medium zucchini (8 ounces), cut into ½-inch cubes

2 baby Italian eggplants (5 ounces each), cut into ½-inch cubes

2 plum tomatoes, cut into ½-inch cubes

DIRECTIONS

Step 1. Preheat the oven to 350°F.

Step 2. Place a steamer basket in a sauté pan with water. Add the potato and cook for about 5 minutes or until tender.

Step 3. In a large bowl, beat together the eggs, egg whites, oregano, pepper, Parmesan and feta cheeses; set aside.

Step 4. In a medium ovenproof skillet, heat the olive oil over medium heat. Add the shallot, zucchini and eggplant and cook for 5 minutes. Add the tomatoes and cooked potato, toss together and cook for another 2 minutes.

Step 5. Pour the egg mixture into the pan of vegetables and cook for 3 minutes, or just until the edges start to set. Transfer the skillet to the oven. Bake for 25 to 30 minutes, or until the frittata is puffed and browned. Let stand a few minutes before cutting.

Arugula Salad

Prep Time: 10 minutes
Cook Time: None
Serves: 2

INGREDIENTS

4 cups arugula

2 radishes, thinly sliced

1 small cucumber, thinly sliced

1 tablespoon chopped black olives

2 tablespoons walnuts

4 tablespoons Berry Balsamic Dressing (page 281)

DIRECTIONS

Step 1. In a large bowl, place the arugula, radishes and cucumber. Top with the olives and walnuts and drizzle with the dressing.

Hummus Veggie Wrap

Prep Time: 5 minutes

Cook Time: None

Yield: 1½ cups

Servings: 12 (2 tablespoons per serving)

INGREDIENTS FOR HUMMUS

1 can chickpeas, well drained

3 tablespoons tahini

5 tablespoons freshly squeezed lemon juice

1 tablespoon extra-virgin olive oil

1 tablespoon water

1 tablespoon finely chopped fresh parsley or 1 teaspoon dried parsley

Pinch of sea salt

DIRECTIONS

Step 1. Place all of the ingredients in the bowl of a food processor and puree until smooth. Adjust the consistency if desired with additional water or lemon juice.

INGREDIENTS FOR WRAP

Wrap: 2 large Boston, romaine or green leaf lettuce leaves, washed and patted dry *or* 2 nori sheets *or* 2 Paleo Wraps

Veggies: ¾ cup vegetables: shredded carrots, sliced cucumbers, chopped tomatoes, radishes, etc.

Healthy Fats: ¼ avocado and 1 tablespoon Lemon Dill Dressing (page 282)

DIRECTIONS

Step 1. Fill each wrap with 2 tablespoons hummus. Top with all of the other ingredients. Then drizzle with the dressing.

Swift Tips

- Hummus lends itself to many flavorful variations, so play around with the basic recipe and enjoy!
- Hummus with a Hint of Heat: Add ½ cup roasted red pepper and substitute ¼ teaspoon cayenne pepper for the parsley.
- Hummus with a Hint of Sweet: Add 1 small cooked sweet potato and substitute 1 teaspoon garam masala for the parsley.
- Hummus with a Hint of Mint: Substitute 1 tablespoon chopped fresh mint or 1 teaspoon dried mint for the parsley.

Kale Salad with Orange Zinger Chicken

Prep Time: 10 minutes
Cook Time: None
Serves: 2

INGREDIENTS

4 cups shredded kale
1 cup grated carrots
6 ounces grilled boneless chicken breast, sliced (cooked ahead)
2 tablespoons pumpkin seeds
4 tablespoons Orange Zinger Dressing (page 283)

DIRECTIONS

Step 1. In a large bowl, place the kale and carrots. Top with the chicken and pumpkin seeds and drizzle with the dressing.

Lauren's Lentil Soup

Prep Time: 15 minutes
Cook Time: 45 minutes
Serves: 8 (1½ cups per serving)

INGREDIENTS

2 cups dried lentils
9 cups water
1 onion, diced
½ fennel bulb, diced
2 large carrots, diced
2 stalks celery, diced
2 cloves garlic, minced
1 bay leaf
1 teaspoon dried oregano
2 teaspoons garam masala
1 14½-ounce can crushed tomatoes
1 teaspoon red wine vinegar
2 cups chopped fresh spinach or 1 10-ounce package frozen spinach, thawed and drained
Sea salt and freshly ground black pepper to taste

DIRECTIONS

Step 1. Rinse the lentils under running water and pick through them to remove any bits of soil or rocks.

Step 2. In an 8-quart stockpot over medium-high heat, add 1 cup of the water.

Add the onion, fennel, carrots and celery and cook for about 5 minutes, until the vegetables are tender.

Step 3. Stir in the garlic, bay leaf, oregano and garam masala and cook for 2 minutes.

Step 4. Stir in remaining 8 cups of water, the lentils and tomatoes and bring to a boil. Reduce heat to medium and add the vinegar. Simmer for about 35 minutes, or until the lentils are tender. Remove and discard the bay leaf.

Step 5. Add the spinach and cook for an additional 2 to 3 minutes.

Step 6. Add a pinch of sea salt and freshly ground black pepper to taste.

Quinoa Lentil Tabouli with Olive Herbed Pesto

Prep Time: 15 minutes
Cook Time: 20 minutes
Serves: 3

INGREDIENTS

½ cup quinoa, rinsed and soaked

1 cup water

1 14½-ounce can lentils, drained

2 tablespoons Olive Herbed Pesto (page 247)

1 small cucumber, diced

4 plum tomatoes, diced

1 carrot, diced

3 cups mesclun greens

DIRECTIONS

Step 1. In a small saucepan, place the quinoa and water. Bring to a boil over high heat, then reduce the heat to medium-low and simmer for about 15 minutes, until the quinoa is tender. Set aside to cool.

Step 2. Mix the cooled quinoa and lentils with the pesto. Add in cucumber, tomato and carrot.

Step 3. Serve over the greens.

Olive Herbed Pesto

Prep Time: 5 minutes
Cook Time: None
Serves: 6 (2 tablespoons per serving)

INGREDIENTS

½ cup fresh herbs, cleaned and loosely packed (basil, parsley, mint, cilantro, etc.)
2 tablespoons extra-virgin olive oil
2 tablespoons pitted olives
1 tablespoon miso
2 tablespoons freshly squeezed lemon juice
2 tablespoons water
½ teaspoon ground turmeric

DIRECTIONS

Step 1. Place all of the ingredients in a blender or in the bowl of a small food processor and process until smooth.

Swift Tips

- Any remaining pesto can be stored in an airtight container in the refrigerator for up to 5 days.
- The tabouli can also be made with buckwheat groats, a gluten-free, magnesium-rich, alkalinizing food that offers a denser tabouli texture.

Savory Salmon Cakes with Pink Sauerkraut

Prep Time: 10 minutes
Cook Time: 10 minutes
Serves: 4

INGREDIENTS

2 6-ounce cans wild salmon, drained
2 large eggs, beaten
3 tablespoons chopped fresh chives
2 tablespoons finely chopped shallots
½ teaspoon dry mustard
1 teaspoon dried dill
½ cup almond flour
2 teaspoons extra-virgin olive oil

DIRECTIONS

Step 1. In a medium bowl, combine the salmon, eggs, chives, shallots, dry mustard, dill and flour. Form the salmon mixture into 4 equal-sized patties.

Step 2. In a large skillet over medium-high heat, add the olive oil and place the patties in the pan. Brown the patties on one side, flip over and cook until done (about 10 minutes total).

Step 3. Serve topped with 2 tablespoons Yogurt Chive Dressing (page 284) and Pink Sauerkraut, made ahead (page see below).

Pink Sauerkraut

Prep Time: 15 minutes
Fermenting Time: 7 to 14 days
Yield: 12 cups

INGREDIENTS

1½ tablespoons pickling sea salt (this is a fine sea salt)

1 quart water

1 small head of green cabbage, shredded

1 small head of red cabbage, shredded

1 tablespoon caraway seeds

DIRECTIONS

Step 1. Make a brine by mixing the salt and water in a clean jar.

Step 2. In a large bowl, combine the cabbage and caraway seeds. Pack the mixture into a separate, 1-quart mason jar. Keep packing the cabbage down using a wooden spoon.

Step 3. Fill the jar with brine to 1 inch below the rim. Top with a "plug" slightly smaller than the opening of the container to keep the vegetables packed tightly in the jar. (I find that a sliced daikon radish works well).

Step 4. Tighten the lid on the jar, mark the date, and place in cool area (65 to 70°F) and allow to ferment, checking the fermentation progress every 2 days.

Step 5. To check the fermentation progress: Hold the jar over the sink and carefully open the lid. You may notice expansion of air from the fermentation process. Skim the surface of foam/scum, if necessary. Refill with additional brine to 1 inch below the rim of the jar. Retighten the jar lid and place in a cool area. Continue to check the sauerkraut every other day until you don't see bubbles rising in the jar, which means the fermentation process is complete. This usually takes between 7 and 14 days.

Step 6. Store in the refrigerator for up to 6 months.

Southwestern Salad with Avocado Cream Dressing

Prep Time: 15 minutes

Cook Time: None

Serves: 2

INGREDIENTS

1 head of romaine lettuce, outer leaves and core removed, cut into
½-inch pieces

2 medium tomatoes, chopped

1 small bunch fresh cilantro, chopped

1 cup cooked black beans

2 tablespoons green chilies

2 tablespoons Avocado Cream Dressing (page 280)

DIRECTIONS

Step 1. In a large bowl, place the lettuce, tomatoes and cilantro. Top with the black beans and chilies and drizzle with the dressing.

Spinach Salad with Basil Balsamic Salmon

Prep Time: 5 minutes

Cook Time: None

Serves: 2

INGREDIENTS

4 cups baby spinach, washed

1 medium red bell pepper, sliced

3 radishes, thinly sliced

6 ounces wild salmon, freshly cooked or canned

2 tablespoons sunflower seeds

4 tablespoons Basil Balsamic Dressing (page 281)

DIRECTIONS

Step 1. In a large bowl, place the spinach, bell pepper and radishes. Top with the salmon and sunflower seeds and drizzle with the dressing.

Turkey Burger Vegetable Soup

Prep Time: 15 minutes

Cook Time: 30 minutes

Serves: 8 (1½ cups per serving)

INGREDIENTS

3 cups water

1 yellow bell pepper, diced

1 red bell pepper, diced

1 green bell pepper, diced

4 carrots, diced

1 small fennel bulb, diced

2 pounds lean ground turkey

1 14½-ounce can diced tomatoes

5 red or purple potatoes, diced into 1-inch cubes

2 cups shredded green cabbage

3 tablespoons tomato paste

½ teaspoon sea salt

½ teaspoon freshly ground black pepper

2 teaspoons dried parsley flakes

½ teaspoon dried oregano

¼ teaspoon cayenne pepper

DIRECTIONS

Step 1. In a large pot over medium-high heat, add 1 cup of the water. Add the peppers, carrots and fennel and cook for about 5 minutes, until al dente.

Step 2. Add the ground turkey to the vegetables and cook for about 8 minutes, until the turkey is no longer pink.

Step 3. Add the remaining 2 cups of water, the tomatoes, potatoes, cabbage, tomato paste, salt, pepper, parsley, oregano and cayenne. Stir to combine, then bring to a boil.

Step 4. Reduce the heat to low, then cover the pot and simmer the soup for 15 to 20 minutes, until the potatoes are tender but not mushy.

Swift Tip

- *Mirepoix* is the French word for a combination of aromatic vegetables used to flavor soups, stews and sauces. A low-FODMAP mirepoix with a combo of peppers, fennel and carrots is used in soup recipes in Weeks 1 and 2. If FODMAPs are friendly to your digestive system, go ahead and substitute the flavorful trio of the higher FODMAPs: garlic, onions and celery.

Unclassic Chicken Waldorf Salad

Prep Time: 10 minutes
Cook Time: None
Serves: 2

INGREDIENTS

1 medium apple, chopped
1 stalk celery, chopped

1 scallion, chopped, white and green parts

2 tablespoons walnuts

6 ounces skinless baked chicken, sliced or cut in 1-inch pieces

4 cups chopped romaine lettuce

4 tablespoons Yogurt Chive Dressing (page 284)

DIRECTIONS

Step 1. Place all of the ingredients in a medium bowl and toss until well coated.

Wrapped Fish with Veggies and Lemon Dill Dressing

Prep Time: 5 minutes

Cook Time: None

Serves: 1 (2 wraps)

INGREDIENTS FOR WRAP

Wrap: 2 large Boston, romaine or green leaf lettuce leaves, washed and patted dry *or* 2 nori sheets *or* 2 Paleo Wraps

Fish: 3 ounces skipjack tuna or sardines, water-packed

Veggies: ¾ cup vegetables: shredded carrots, sliced cucumbers, chopped tomatoes, thinly sliced radishes, sprouts

Healthy Fats: 1 tablespoon chopped olives and 1 tablespoon Lemon Dill Dressing (page 282)

DIRECTIONS

Step 1. Fill the wraps with all of the ingredients, drizzle with the dressing and enjoy.

The Swift Menu Plan: Dinners

Dinner is the reassuring ritual that signals the end of the day, whether it's convivial and social or a meditative quiet time. No matter how you slice it, dinner is about feeding our bodies with good healthy food, the culmination of a nourishing day.

Basil Balsamic Baked Chicken with Italian Herbed Zucchini

Prep Time: 5 minutes
Cook Time: 45 minutes
Serves: 4

INGREDIENTS

2 bone-in, skin-on, split chicken breasts
½ cup Basil Balsamic Dressing (page 281)

DIRECTIONS

Step 1. Preheat the oven to 325°F.

Step 2. Remove the excess fat and excess skin from the chicken (do not remove the skin; just cut off any hanging flaps), wash, pat dry and set aside.

Step 3. In a large shallow baking dish, add the chicken and well-whisked marinade until the chicken is well coated.

Step 4. Cover the dish with a lid or aluminum foil and bake for 30 minutes.

Step 5. Remove the lid or foil and bake for an additional 15 minutes, or until the juices run clear or a thermometer inserted into the thickest part of the breast, not touching the bone, reads 165°F.

Step 6. Remove the skin before serving.

Italian Herbed Zucchini

Prep Time: 3 minutes

Cook Time: 20 minutes

Serves: 4

INGREDIENTS

4 medium zucchini, cut into 1-inch cubes

2 tablespoons extra-virgin olive oil

2 teaspoons dried oregano

2 teaspoons crushed rosemary

1 28-ounce can tomatoes, diced

DIRECTIONS

Step 1. Preheat the oven to 325°F.

Step 2. Toss the zucchini lightly with the olive oil, oregano, rosemary and tomatoes.

Step 3. Place the zucchini in a small baking dish and bake for 20 minutes. (You can bake this and the Basil Balsamic Chicken [page 254] at the same time.)

Swift Tip

- Make the dressing ahead of time and store in a glass jar with a lid in the refrigerator until ready to use. Marinate your chicken breasts in the morning, then cover and refrigerate until ready to cook.

Citrus Glazed Maple Salmon with Pineapple Cabbage Slaw

Prep Time: 15 minutes

Cook Time: 10 minutes

Serves: 4

INGREDIENTS

¼ cup freshly squeezed lemon juice

1 teaspoon orange zest

1 teaspoon grated fresh ginger or ½ teaspoon ground ginger

1 tablespoon 100 percent pure maple syrup

½ cup gluten-free tamari

1 pound wild salmon fillets

DIRECTIONS

Step 1. Preheat the oven to 350°F.

Step 2. In a glass measuring container, place the lemon juice, orange zest, ginger, maple syrup and tamari. Whisk until blended.

Step 3. Rinse the salmon and place it skin-side down in a glass baking dish. Pour the marinade over the fish, cover and bake for about 10 minutes, or until the salmon flakes.

Pineapple Cabbage Slaw with Mint Tahini Dressing

Prep Time: 10 minutes

Cook Time: None

Serves: 4 (1½ cups per serving)

INGREDIENTS

6 cups finely shredded cabbage

½ cup chopped celery

6 radishes, chopped

4 scallions (green part only), diced

1 cup chopped fresh pineapple

¼ cup slivered almonds

½ cup Mint Tahini Dressing (page 282)

DIRECTIONS

Step 1. In a large bowl, combine all of the ingredients.

Step 2. Pour the dressing over the salad and toss together until coated.

Swift Tip

- You can substitute the Pink Sauerkraut (page 248) for the pineapple cabbage slaw for a fermented food boost.

Herbes de Provence Chicken with Roasted Vegetables

Prep Time: 5 minutes
Cook Time: 30 minutes
Serves: 4

INGREDIENTS

1 pound boneless, skinless chicken breasts

1½ tablespoons extra-virgin olive oil

1 tablespoon Herbes de Provence

DIRECTIONS

Step 1. Preheat the oven to 325°F.

Step 2. Place the chicken breasts in a shallow baking dish.

Step 3. Coat the chicken with the olive oil and sprinkle the herb mixture evenly over the chicken.

Step 4. Bake for about 30 minutes, until chicken is cooked through. A meat thermometer should read 165°F when the chicken is done.

Roasted Vegetables

Prep Time: 10 minutes
Cook Time: 30 minutes
Serves: 4

INGREDIENTS

1 pound purple potatoes, unpeeled

3 parsnips, unpeeled

3 turnips, unpeeled

2 tablespoons extra-virgin olive oil

3 tablespoons freshly chopped parsley or 1 tablespoon dried parsley

DIRECTIONS

Step 1. Preheat the oven to 325°F.

Step 2. Wash the potatoes, parsnips and turnips thoroughly and cut into 1-inch cubes.

Step 3. Place the vegetables in a baking dish and toss with the olive oil and parsley until evenly coated.

Step 4. Bake for about 30 minutes, or until the vegetables are tender.

Swift Tips

- The stems and skins of vegetables and fruits are jam-packed with phytonutrients and micronutrients, so include them in as many meals as you can, vegetables especially.
- Double this recipe so you have delicious veggies on hand!

Lemon Dill Shrimp with Sesame Bok Choy

Prep Time: 10 minutes
Cook Time: 5 minutes
Serves: 4

INGREDIENTS

1 pound medium shrimp
1 cup Lemon Dill Dressing (page 282)

DIRECTIONS

Step 1. Peel and devein the shrimp.

Step 2. In a medium bowl, coat the shrimp with the dressing mixture.

Step 3. In a medium skillet, sauté the shrimp on medium-high heat for about 4 minutes, until they are pink and opaque throughout.

Sesame Bok Choy

Prep Time: 5 minutes
Cook Time: 5 minutes
Serves: 4

INGREDIENTS

1 pound bok choy, chopped in strips

1 medium red bell pepper, sliced

1 teaspoon sesame seeds

DIRECTIONS

Step 1. Add the bok choy and bell pepper to a steamer basket with water in a stainless-steel skillet.

Step 2. Cover and steam for 3 minutes, then remove from the steamer and top with the sesame seeds.

Moroccan Eggplant

Prep Time: 15 minutes

Cook Time: 30 minutes

Serves: 4

INGREDIENTS

1 tablespoon extra-virgin olive oil

1 large onion, cut in half and thinly sliced

3 cloves garlic, finely chopped

1 medium red bell pepper, cut in 1-inch squares

1 medium eggplant, cut into 1-inch cubes

1 teaspoon garam masala

1¼ cups vegetable broth

½ cup tomato sauce

1 15-ounce can garbanzo beans, rinsed and drained

½ cup raisins

Sea salt and freshly ground black pepper to taste

1 tablespoon chopped fresh cilantro

DIRECTIONS

Step 1. Heat 1 tablespoon olive oil in Dutch oven over medium heat; add the onion and cook for about 5 minutes, stirring frequently, until the onion is translucent.

Step 2. Add the garlic, bell pepper, eggplant and garam masala. Stir to mix well and cook for 3 minutes.

Step 3. Add broth and tomato sauce. Stir again to mix, cover, reduce the heat to medium-low and cook for about 15 minutes, stirring occasionally, or until the peppers and eggplant are tender.

Step 4. Add garbanzo beans and raisins. Simmer for another 5 minutes. Season with salt and pepper. Top with chopped cilantro.

Step 5. Serve with ½ cup steamed quinoa, brown rice or buckwheat groats (kasha) prepared according to the package directions.

Swift Tip

- The health-promoting properties of garlic and onions are released if you let them sit for a few minutes after peeled and sliced.

Orange Zinger Cod with Spinach and Cherry Tomatoes

Prep Time: 10 minutes
Cook Time: 20 minutes
Serves: 4

INGREDIENTS

¼ cup Orange Zinger Dressing (page 283)
½ cup Kalamata olives, pitted
½ cup coarsely chopped fresh parsley

4 wild cod fillets (4 to 6 ounces each) or other wild fish

2 teaspoons extra-virgin olive oil

DIRECTIONS

Step 1. Preheat oven to 350°F.

Step 2. In the bowl of a food processor, combine the dressing, olives and parsley and blend until it resembles a smooth paste.

Step 3. Place the fish in a lightly oiled baking dish. Spread 1 tablespoon of the olive pesto onto each fish fillet.

Step 4. Bake for about 20 minutes, until the fish is flaky, and serve with Spinach with Cherry Tomatoes (see below).

Spinach with Cherry Tomatoes

Prep Time: 5 minutes
Cook Time: 3 minutes
Serves: 4

INGREDIENTS

8 cups fresh spinach leaves
1 cup cherry tomatoes, halved
Pinch of sea salt (optional)

DIRECTIONS

Step 1. Place a steamer basket in a medium saucepan with water.

Step 2. Add the spinach and cherry tomatoes, cover and steam for 2 minutes.

Pecan-Crusted Chicken with Swiss Chard and Orange-Scented Carrots

Prep Time: 5 minutes

Cook Time: 10 minutes

Serves: 4

INGREDIENTS

4 boneless, skinless chicken breasts (4 to 6 ounces each)

¼ cup chopped fresh parsley

½ tablespoon dried rosemary

¼ cup crushed pecans

1 tablespoon Dijon mustard

Pinch of sea salt (optional)

1 tablespoon extra-virgin coconut oil

DIRECTIONS

Step 1. Place each chicken breast on a cutting board and cover with wax paper; pound firmly with a meat mallet to flatten slightly.

Step 2. In a small bowl, mix together the parsley, rosemary and pecans and sprinkle the on a plate.

Step 3. Brush both sides of each chicken breast with a thin layer of Dijon mustard and then dip into the herb mixture so that both sides are coated.

Step 4. In a sauté pan, heat the coconut oil over medium heat. Add the chicken and sauté for about 5 minutes on one side. Turn the chicken over and cook for about 5 minutes more, until cooked through. Remove from the pan and set aside.

Swiss Chard

Prep Time: 10 minutes

Cook Time: 4 minutes

Serves: 4

INGREDIENTS

2 tablespoons extra-virgin olive oil

Freshly squeezed juice of 1 lemon

8 cups Swiss chard

2 cups water

Red pepper flakes (optional)

Pinch of sea salt (optional)

DIRECTIONS

Step 1. In a glass measuring container, whisk together the olive oil and lemon juice.

Step 2. Tear the chard into 2- or 3-inch pieces. Place a steamer basket in a sauté pan with water. Add the chard, cover and cook about 4 minutes, until the greens wilt.

Step 3. Remove the chard from the steamer basket and drain any excess water.

Step 4. Drizzle the lemon–olive oil mixture over the greens and serve. Sprinkle with red pepper flakes and sea salt if desired.

Orange-Scented Carrots

Prep Time: 5 minutes
Cook Time: 8 minutes
Serves: 4

INGREDIENTS

½ pound carrots
½ teaspoon dried basil
1 teaspoon freshly grated orange peel (from 1 small organic orange)
   or ½ teaspoon dried orange peel

DIRECTIONS

Step 1. Wash the carrots and cut them into ¼-inch slices.

Step 2. Place a steamer basket in a sauté pan with water. Add the carrots, cover and cook until they are al dente.

Step 3. Remove the carrots from steamer and drain.

Step 4. Sprinkle the carrots with basil and orange peel.

Pesto Chicken on Bean Pasta with Sautéed Kale

Prep Time: 5 minutes
Cook Time: 10 minutes
Serves: 4

INGREDIENTS

1 pound boneless, skinless chicken breasts
3 tablespoons extra-virgin olive oil
¼ cup walnuts

2 cups fresh parsley

2 teaspoons Dijon mustard

2 teaspoons freshly squeezed lemon juice

Pinch of sea salt (optional)

DIRECTIONS

Step 1. Place each chicken breast on a cutting board and cover with wax paper; pound firmly with a meat mallet to flatten slightly. Slice into thin strips.

Step 2. In a sauté pan, heat 1 tablespoon of the olive oil over medium heat. Add the chicken and sauté for 5 minutes on one side. Turn the chicken over and cook for another 5 minutes, until cooked through. Remove the chicken from the pan and set aside.

Step 3. In the bowl of a food processor, place the walnuts, parsley, mustard, lemon juice and the 2 remaining tablespoons of olive oil and process until desired pesto consistency is obtained.

Step 4. Toss the chicken in the pesto, add a pinch of salt if desired, and serve with bean pasta and Sautéed Kale (see below).

Sautéed Kale

Prep Time: 5 minutes

Cook Time: 4 minutes

Serves: 4

INGREDIENTS

1½ pounds lacinato kale, stems and leaves coarsely chopped

1 tablespoon extra-virgin olive oil

2 teaspoons freshly squeezed lemon juice

Red pepper flakes (optional)

DIRECTIONS

Step 1. Place a steamer basket in a sauté pan with water. Add the kale, cover and cook for about 4 minutes, or until the leaves are softened.

Step 2. Remove the kale, drain and place in a bowl. Drizzle with olive oil, lemon juice and red pepper flakes if using.

Swift Tip

- You don't need to swear off pasta anymore! Delicious "bean pastas," high in protein and fiber, are now available in the marketplace. Explore Asian is one of my favorite brands!

Simple Grilled Fish with Zesty Sesame Broccoli

Prep Time: 5 minutes
Cook Time: 8 to 10 minutes
Serves: 4

INGREDIENTS

1 pound wild-caught white fish, skin off
1 tablespoon extra-virgin olive oil
Herbal seasoning of choice

DIRECTIONS

Step 1. Brush the fish with olive oil and sprinkle with herbal seasoning.

Step 2. Cook on a grill or hot grill pan for 4 to 5 minutes each side, based on a ¾-inch-thick fish, or until the fish flakes.

Zesty Sesame Broccoli

Prep Time: 5 minutes
Cook Time: 6 minutes
Serves: 4

INGREDIENTS

1 head of broccoli, washed and cut into florets
1 tablespoon extra-virgin olive oil
2 teaspoons toasted black sesame seeds
1 teaspoon freshly grated lemon zest

DIRECTIONS

Step 1. Place a steamer basket in a sauté pan with water. Add the broccoli, cover and steam for 6 to 8 minutes or until al dente.

Step 2. Remove the broccoli, drain and place in a medium-size bowl.

Step 3. Drizzle the broccoli with olive oil and sprinkle with sesame seeds and lemon zest. Toss and serve.

Slow Cooker Beef Stew

Prep Time: 10 minutes
Cook Time: 4 to 12 hours, depending on the heat setting
Serves: 4

INGREDIENTS

1 pound grass-fed tenderloin or sirloin beef, cut into 1-inch cubes
1 medium onion, diced
2 sweet potatoes, unpeeled, cut into 1-inch cubes
4 carrots, cut into 1-inch cubes

2 stalks celery, diced

1 medium parsnip, cut into 1-inch cubes

1 cup sliced portobello mushrooms

1 clove garlic, minced

1 tablespoon gluten-free Worcestershire sauce

½ teaspoon sea salt

½ teaspoon freshly ground black pepper

2 bay leaves or 1 teaspoon crushed bay leaf

2 teaspoons dried rosemary

2 teaspoons dried parsley

2½ cups cold water

DIRECTIONS

Step 1. Place all of the ingredients in a slow cooker.

Step 2. Cook for 10 to 12 hours on low or 4 to 6 hours on high.

Slow Cooker Coconut Curry Chicken

Prep Time: 15 minutes

Slow Cooker Time: 4 to 5 hours

Serves: 4

INGREDIENTS

1 cup Swift and Simple Additive-free Homemade Coconut Milk (page 236)

3 cups low-sodium vegetable stock

8 chicken thighs, skinned, or 1 pound gluten-free tempeh, cut into 1-inch chunks

1 medium onion, sliced

3 cloves garlic, sliced

1 red bell pepper, sliced

2 zucchini, cut into 1-inch chunks

1 cup cauliflower florets

2 medium sweet potatoes, diced into ½-inch cubes

1 1-inch piece of fresh ginger, coarsely chopped

2 tablespoons gluten-free tamari

1 teaspoon garam masala

1 teaspoon ground turmeric

DIRECTIONS

Step 1. Pour the coconut milk and vegetable stock into a slow cooker.

Step 2. Add the remaining ingredients in the order listed.

Step 3. Cover and cook on low for 4 to 5 hours.

Swift Nutty Fish with Lemon Asparagus

Prep Time: 5 minutes

Cook Time: 15 minutes

Serves: 4

INGREDIENTS

¼ cup chopped macadamia nuts

Freshly grated zest of 1 lemon or lime

1 pound wild white fish, such as sole, halibut or tilapia

Sea salt and freshly ground pepper to taste

1 tablespoon extra-virgin olive oil

DIRECTIONS

Step 1. Preheat oven to 350°F.

Step 2. In a small mixing bowl, combine the macadamia nuts and zest and set aside.

Step 3. Place the fish on a baking sheet and season with salt and pepper to taste. Drizzle with olive oil and the nutty zest topping.

Step 4. Place the fish in the oven and cook for about 15 minutes, or until the flesh is flaky.

Lemon Asparagus

Prep Time: 2 minutes
Cook Time: 20 minutes
Serves: 4

INGREDIENTS

1 bunch of asparagus, with spears as thin as possible
2 tablespoons extra-virgin olive oil
1 teaspoon freshly grated lemon zest
Sea salt and freshly ground black pepper to taste

DIRECTIONS

Step 1. Preheat oven to 350°F.

Step 2. Trim the bottom of the asparagus and wash thoroughly.

Step 3. Place the asparagus in a baking dish. Drizzle with olive oil. Sprinkle with the lemon zest, and salt and pepper to taste.

Step 4. Bake for about 20 minutes, until tender.

Taco Skillet Pie

Prep Time: 5 minutes
Cook Time: 20 minutes
Serves: 4

INGREDIENTS

1 tablespoon extra-virgin olive oil

1 pound lean ground turkey

1 19-ounce can black beans, drained

1 14½-ounce can petite cut fire-roasted tomatoes

1 4½-ounce can green chilies

1 tablespoon ground cumin

½ log organic cooked polenta, sliced into ½-inch-thick rounds

⅓ cup grated organic cheddar cheese

1 avocado, peeled and diced

DIRECTIONS

Step 1. Preheat the oven to 425°F.

Step 2. In large, ovenproof skillet, heat the olive oil over medium heat. Add the turkey and sauté for about 8 minutes, until no longer pink.

Step 3. Stir in black beans, tomatoes, chilies and cumin. Bring to a boil over high heat and boil for 1 minute.

Step 4. Cover the mixture with the polenta rounds, place in the oven and bake for 10 minutes.

Step 5. Sprinkle top with cheese and continue baking for another 3 minutes, until golden brown. Garnish with the avocado.

Tempeh Vegetable Skewer

Prep Time: 15 minutes and up to 2 hours of marinade time
Cook Time: 10 minutes
Serves: 4

INGREDIENTS

1 red bell pepper, cut into 1-inch squares

1 yellow bell pepper, cut into 1-inch squares

1 orange bell pepper, cut into 1-inch squares

1 medium zucchini, cut into ½-inch sections

16 cherry tomatoes

1 cup fresh pineapple, cut into 1-inch cubes

1 8-ounce package organic gluten-free tempeh, cut into 1-inch
squares

¼ cup extra-virgin olive oil

¼ cup freshly squeezed lemon juice

½ teaspoon Chinese five-spice

8 wooden or metal skewers (soak wooden skewers in a pan of water,
fully submerged, for a minimum of 20 minutes)

DIRECTIONS

Step 1. In a large bowl, combine the bell peppers, zucchini, tomatoes, pineapple and tempeh.

Step 2. In a separate glass container, whisk together the olive oil, lemon juice and Chinese five-spice.

Step 3. Pour the marinade over the vegetables and stir to coat. Marinate in the refrigerator for 1 to 2 hours.

Step 4. Preheat the grill to medium high, or you can use the broiler in the oven.

Step 5. Place the vegetables, pineapple and tempeh on the skewers in an alternating fashion.

Step 6. Place skewers on the preheated grill, turning onto all 4 sides until done, approximately 10 minutes.

Swift Tip

- Take advantage of fresh produce in season, and if the FODMAP "gang" isn't problematic for you, add some onions and mushrooms to the skewers.

Thai Vegetable Stir-Fry with Shrimp

Prep Time: 20 minutes

Cook Time: 6 minutes

Serves: 4

INGREDIENTS

1 tablespoon extra-virgin coconut oil

3 carrots, cut on the diagonal

1 red bell pepper, sliced into strips

3 cups sliced bok choy

4 scallions (green part only), thinly sliced on the diagonal

1 pound large shrimp, peeled and deveined

1 cup fresh bean sprouts

¼ cup freshly squeezed lime juice

2 tablespoons gluten-free tamari

1 teaspoon grated fresh ginger or ½ teaspoon ground ginger

2 teaspoons toasted sesame oil

¼ cup chopped fresh basil

1 tablespoon sesame seeds

DIRECTIONS

Step 1. In a large saucepan or wok, heat the coconut oil over medium-high heat.

Step 2. Add the carrots and bell pepper and stir-fry for 2 minutes.

Step 3. Add the bok choy, scallions and shrimp and cook for 2 minutes more.

Step 4. Add the bean sprouts, lime juice, tamari, ginger and sesame oil and cook for an additional 2 minutes.

Step 5. Toss with the basil and sesame seeds just before serving.

Swift Tip

- You can substitute tempeh for the shrimp for a fermented food boost. Be sure to purchase a brand that is certified gluten-free.

Turkey Cutlets with Kiwi Salsa, Green Beans Almondine, In-Skin Baked Potato and Lemon Dill Dressing

Prep Time: 15 minutes

Cook Time: 6 minutes

Serves: 4

INGREDIENTS

3 kiwis, peeled and chopped

2 teaspoons freshly squeezed lime juice (juice from ½ lime)

1 teaspoon grated fresh ginger or ½ teaspoon ground ginger

1 tablespoon chopped fresh mint or 1 teaspoon dried mint

4 turkey breast cutlets (4 ounces each, about ½ inch thick)

1 tablespoon coconut oil

Pinch of sea salt

Freshly ground black pepper to taste

DIRECTIONS

Step 1. In a bowl, combine the kiwi, lime juice, ginger and mint. Set the kiwi salsa aside.

Step 2. Preheat a grill pan to medium. Coat both sides of the turkey with coconut oil and season with salt and pepper. Grill the turkey for 3 minutes on one side, then turn over and cook for about 3 minutes, or until cooked through.

Step 3. Serve topped with the kiwi salsa.

Green Beans Almondine

Prep Time: 10 minutes
Cook Time: 6 minutes
Serves: 4

INGREDIENTS

1 tablespoon extra-virgin olive oil
¼ cup slivered almonds
1 pound green beans, trimmed, or 12 ounces frozen green beans
½ red bell pepper, cut into thin strips

DIRECTIONS

Step 1. In a medium sauté pan, heat the olive oil over medium-low heat. Add the almonds and cook for 1 to 2 minutes, stirring occasionally, until lightly browned.

Step 2. Add the green beans and bell pepper and cook for 5 minutes, stirring occasionally.

Enjoy with a medium baked potato with 1 tablespoon Lemon Dill Dressing (page 282). If oven baked, it will take 45 minutes at 350°F. Be sure to pierce the potato skin before baking.

Turkey Sun-dried Tomato Meat Loaf with Roasted Red Rosemary Potatoes

Prep Time: 15 minutes
Cook Time: 50 minutes
Serves: 8

INGREDIENTS

2 large eggs

½ cup almond flour

2 pounds lean ground turkey

1 red bell pepper, chopped

2 celery stalks, chopped

2 scallions, green part only, chopped

¼ cup diced, rehydrated and drained sun-dried tomatoes

1 10-ounce package frozen spinach, thawed and drained

¼ cup tomato paste

2 tablespoons gluten-free tamari

2 teaspoons dried sage

2 teaspoons dry mustard

1 teaspoon freshly ground black pepper

DIRECTIONS

Step 1. Preheat oven to 350°F.

Step 2. In a large mixing bowl, whisk the eggs.

Step 3. Add the almond flour to the eggs and stir until blended.

Step 4. Add the turkey, bell pepper, celery, scallions, sun-dried tomatoes, spinach, tomato paste, tamari, sage, dry mustard, and pepper and mix until blended together.

Step 5. Place the turkey mixture in a lightly oiled 9 x 13-inch baking dish.

Step 6. Bake for 50 minutes, or until a meat thermometer inserted in the center reads 165°F. (Note: When removed from oven, the meat loaf will have a slight milky appearance.)

Roasted Red Rosemary Potatoes

Prep Time: 10 minutes
Cook Time: 35 minutes
Serves: 4

INGREDIENTS

1½ pounds red or purple potatoes, washed, unpeeled and cut into
   quarters
1 tablespoon extra-virgin olive oil
2 tablespoons minced fresh parsley
1 teaspoon crushed rosemary
Sea salt and freshly ground pepper to taste

DIRECTIONS

Step 1. Preheat the oven to 350°F.

Step 2. Place the potatoes in an 8 x 8-inch baking dish.

Step 3. Coat the potatoes with the olive oil.

Step 4. Add the parsley, rosemary, salt and pepper to taste.

Step 5. Bake covered for 25 minutes and uncovered an additional 10 minutes, until golden brown.

Vietnamese Beef and Green Beans

Prep Time: 15 minutes
Cook Time: 12 minutes
Serves: 4

INGREDIENTS

2 teaspoons arrowroot powder

2 tablespoons brown rice vinegar

1 teaspoon toasted sesame oil

2 tablespoons grated fresh ginger or 2 teaspoons ground ginger

2 tablespoons gluten-free tamari

1 pound flank or flatiron steak, cut into ¼-inch-thick slices

1 tablespoon extra-virgin coconut oil

1 pound green beans, trimmed and sliced on the diagonal into 2-inch pieces

1 red bell pepper, sliced lengthwise into ¼-inch pieces

2 scallions (green tops only), cut on the diagonal into ½-inch pieces

¼ cup water

¼ teaspoon red pepper flakes (optional)

DIRECTIONS

Step 1. Marinate the beef: In a medium bowl, whisk together the arrowroot, vinegar, oil, ginger and 1 tablespoon of the tamari until the arrowroot is well dissolved.

Step 2. Add the beef and toss to coat. Cover and place in refrigerator to marinate for 10 minutes.

Step 3. Heat a wok or large skillet over high heat until a bead of water sizzles and evaporates on contact. Add the coconut oil and swirl gently to coat the bottom. Add the beef and stir-fry for 4 minutes. Transfer to a plate and set aside.

Step 4. In the same wok, add green beans, bell pepper and scallions and cook for 2 minutes.

Step 5. Add the water and cover with a lid. Allow the vegetables to steam for 3 to 4 minutes, or until they are crisp-tender.

Step 6. Return the beef to the wok, add the remaining 1 tablespoon of tamari and heat for 1 minute.

Step 7. Sprinkle with red pepper flakes if desired.

Step 8. Serve with ½ cup steamed black (or brown) rice cooked according to the package directions.

Dressings

Avocado Cream Dressing

Prep Time: 5 minutes
Cook Time: None
Serves: 8 (2 tablespoons per serving)

INGREDIENTS

¼ cup freshly squeezed lime juice

¼ cup water

1 tablespoon extra-virgin olive oil

¼ teaspoon chipotle chili powder

1 avocado, peeled and pitted

DIRECTIONS

Step 1. Place all of the ingredients in the bowl of a small food processor and blend until smooth. Store in the refrigerator.

Basil Balsamic Dressing

Prep Time: 5 minutes

Cook Time: None

Serves: 8 (2 tablespoons per serving)

INGREDIENTS

½ cup extra-virgin olive oil

¼ cup balsamic vinegar

1 tablespoon finely chopped fresh basil or 2 teaspoons dried basil

¼ cup water

DIRECTIONS

Step 1. Whisk together all of the ingredients in a small bowl until well blended.

Berry Balsamic Dressing

Prep Time: 5 minutes

Cook Time: None

Serves: 8 (2 tablespoons per serving)

INGREDIENTS

½ cup extra-virgin olive oil

¼ cup balsamic vinegar

¼ cup fresh or frozen wild blueberries

¼ cup water

DIRECTIONS

Step 1. Blend all of the ingredients in a small bowl.

Lemon Dill Dressing

Prep Time: 5 minutes

Cook Time: None

Serves: 8 (2 tablespoons per serving)

INGREDIENTS

½ cup extra-virgin olive oil

¼ cup freshly squeezed lemon juice

1 teaspoon Dijon mustard

2 tablespoons finely chopped fresh dill or 2 teaspoons dried dill

DIRECTIONS

Step 1. Whisk together all of the ingredients in a small bowl until well blended.

Mint Tahini Dressing

Prep Time: 5 minutes

Cook Time: None

Serves: 12 (2 tablespoons per serving)

INGREDIENTS

½ cup tahini

1 tablespoon extra-virgin olive oil

½ cup freshly squeezed lime juice

¼ cup fresh mint leaves

¼ cup water

DIRECTIONS

Step 1. Add all of the ingredients to the bowl of a small food processor and blend until smooth.

Orange Zinger Dressing

Prep Time: 5 minutes

Cook Time: None

Serves: 6 (2 tablespoons per serving)

INGREDIENTS

½ cup extra-virgin olive oil

2 tablespoons apple cider vinegar

2 tablespoons freshly squeezed orange juice

½ teaspoon freshly grated orange peel (zest of 1 medium orange)

⅛ teaspoon ground cinnamon

DIRECTIONS

Step 1. Whisk together all of the ingredients in a small bowl until well blended.

Peanut Lime Dressing

Prep Time: 5 minutes

Cook Time: None

Serves: 6 (2 tablespoons per serving)

INGREDIENTS

¼ cup natural peanut butter (creamy or crunchy)

3 tablespoons freshly squeezed lime juice

¼ teaspoon ground ginger

¼ cup lukewarm water

DIRECTIONS

Step 1. Place all of the ingredients in the bowl of a small food processor and blend until smooth.

Yogurt Chive Dressing

Prep Time: 1 hour 5 minutes
Cook Time: None
Makes: 2 cups

INGREDIENTS

2 cups plain, unsweetened organic yogurt
1 tablespoon extra-virgin olive oil
2 tablespoons minced chives
1 tablespoon minced fresh dill
½ teaspoon sea salt
½ teaspoon freshly ground black pepper

DIRECTIONS

Step 1. Place the yogurt in a medium bowl and blend in the olive oil, chives, dill, salt and pepper. You can store this in the refrigerator for up to 1 week.

Snacks

These days, it can be tough to find the time to eat well. Instead of having a proper meal, a lot of us wind up grazing or snacking our way through the day. As you have learned, your digestive system needs some downtime—and snacking can be a barrier to weight loss if we're not being mindful of the calories that we're casually consuming.

I advise most of my clients, with or without weight concerns, to break the habit of routinely eating between meals. When a snack may be called for—for instance, a gap of four hours or more between meals, or you need a boost to get through a workout—make it nutrient dense and junk-free. Follow these simple guidelines:

- Make fresh fruit your go-to default snack and carry a serving in your bag.
- Don't get stuck in a rut. Rotate snacks to feed your microbiota a varied diet.
- If you're not actually craving a snack on a particular day, skip it. Snacks are on an as-needed basis.
- Avoid "saving" your snack for after dinner—it's more of a use-it-or-lose-it proposition.
- Pick a snack from the following list of healthy choices:

Weeks 1 and 2 Snack Options

- Fresh fruit in season
- ¼ cup raw unsalted almonds, walnuts, pumpkin seeds or sunflower seeds (feel free to make a mix)
- 3 tablespoons olive tapenade with 1 cup raw veggies
- 10 to 15 olives
- 2 teaspoons raw, unsalted nut butter on a small banana
- 1 ounce dark chocolate, 70 percent or more cacao
- ½ serving Swift Smoothie

Weeks 3 and 4 Snack Options

- Any of the options from Weeks 1 and 2
- 1 cup plain, unsweetened organic kefir with a splash of cinnamon or nutmeg
- ½ cup plain, unsweetened organic yogurt with ½ cup berries
- 2 tablespoons Olive Herbed Pesto (page 247) with 1 cup raw veggies
- 1 tablespoon nut butter with celery
- 3 tablespoons Swift Relief Spread (page 289) or Hummus (page 243) on 5 flax crackers
- Energy bar with real food ingredients: Lärabar, Go Raw, Elemental Superfood Seedbar, or try my Swift Cookie recipe on page 290.

Sweet Indulgence

Who among us doesn't enjoy the taste of something indulgent now and then? The problem is, as with any processed food, most dessert treats for sale at the bakery or the deli are loaded with cheap, nutrient-poor ingredients. And they're bursting with gobs of sugar and flour that stimulate cravings for the next fix.

So what's the answer? I believe the fewer sweets, the better, and no sweets, better still. But I also understand that many people need an occasional treat, so here are my thoughts on how to manage sweets in as healthy a way as possible:

- Commit to jettisoning all processed cookies, cakes, candies, ice cream, etc., from your home. If you didn't make it, it shouldn't be in your house.
- Don't keep any sweet treat that might wind up in your mouth squirreled away, in "reserve" for the kids, unexpected guests or visitors (i.e., Santa Claus, the Tooth Fairy, etc.). They don't need the empty calories either!
- If you really need a dessert for a special occasion, then buy or preferably make it at the last possible minute, and get the leftovers out of the house immediately after serving the last slice, long before the late-night munchies hit.
- Bottom line: don't keep processed sweets in the house (or car or garage or hope chest, for that matter).

Once you've committed to tossing out and *keeping out* processed sweets and desserts, then you can look at sweets in a different light—and enjoy the occasional treat guilt-free and without setting off a sugar binge.

The key to a healthy, indulgent dessert? Wonderful, wholesome, organic ingredients that digest slowly, won't spike blood sugar and insulin levels and won't set you up for a crash. Here are a few sweet additions to the plan. As delicious as they are, take it easy: no more than two servings a week. I call this the Sweet Kripalu Effect. Guests at Kripalu enjoy the delicious meals and look forward to the two dessert nights per week.

Apple Almost Pie

Preheat the oven to 350°F. In a small ramekin or baking dish, layer in ½ cup of chopped apples and toss with ½ teaspoon of chia seeds. Top with a drizzle of maple syrup and allspice or cloves to taste. Top with flaxseed (ground or whole) and bake for about 15 minutes, or until the fruit is softened (but not liquid). Remove from the oven, let stand for 3 minutes and enjoy warm!

Chocolate Coconut "Shake"

In a blender, combine 1 cup plain, unsweetened almond milk, 10 ice cubes and 2 tablespoons unsweetened cocoa powder. Add 1 pitted date plus a pinch of cinnamon and blend until smooth.

Chocolate Nut-Butter Sandwich

Take one small (1 ounce) dark chocolate bar—70 percent or more cacao—and cut it in half width-wise. Smear one half with 1 tablespoon of raw, unsalted almond butter, top with the other half of the chocolate and enjoy!

Chow Bella Chia Pudding

(See the recipe on page 225.)

Fresh Fruit Cup

Enjoy the sweetness of 1 cup seasonal fresh fruit with a sprinkle of your favorite spice and unsweetened coconut flakes; for example, orange wedges with cinnamon, pear with nutmeg, etc.

Perfect Yogurt Parfait

(See the recipe on page 231.)

Sweet Potato Power Cakes Sweet Variations: Maple Walnut Banana; Berry; and Chocolate

(See the recipe on page 232.)

Maple Walnut Banana: Substitute 2 teaspoons pure maple walnut extract for the vanilla and ¾ cup banana puree for the carrot.

Berry: Add 1 cup fresh or frozen berries to the batter.

Chocolate: Add 2 tablespoons unsweetened cocoa powder in place of the ginger and add ¾ cup avocado puree.

Swift Chocolate Avocado Playtime Pudding

Prep Time: 10 minutes
Cook Time: None
Serves: 2

INGREDIENTS

1 ripe avocado

3 dates, pitted

½ cup plain, unsweetened nondairy beverage

2 tablespoons unsweetened cocoa powder

1 teaspoon pure vanilla extract (you can vary this recipe with other pure extracts—maple, orange, almond, etc.)

DIRECTIONS

Step 1. Peel and pit the avocado.

Step 2. In the bowl of a high-speed blender, place the avocado, dates, nondairy beverage, cocoa powder, and vanilla. Process until smooth and creamy.

Step 3. Top with unsweetened shredded coconut, grated orange peel or toasted nuts.

Swift Relief Spread

Prep Time: 5 minutes
Cook Time: None
Serves: 10 (3 tablespoons per serving)

This is a favorite recipe at my digestive health workshops for those participants who have sluggish bowels and need to get things moving. It makes a great spread on vegetables, fresh fruit or gluten-free crackers or as a topping for a gluten-free porridge.

INGREDIENTS

1 cup boiling water

½ cup pitted dates

½ cup pitted prunes

¼ cup ground flaxseed

¼ cup rice bran

1 teaspoon favorite spice (I love cloves or allspice!)

DIRECTIONS

Step 1. Place water, dates and prunes in the bowl of a food processor or blender and process until smooth.

Step 2. Add the flaxseed, rice bran and spice. Pulse until smooth. Add more water if needed for thinner consistency.

Swift and Sweet Trail Mix

1 tablespoon each of the following: Dark chocolate chips; unsulfured dried fruit; raw, unsalted nuts and seeds

---

Swift Cookie

Prep Time: 15 minutes

Cook Time: 15 minutes

Yield: 24 cookies (2 cookies per serving)

INGREDIENTS

¾ cup raw, unsalted almond butter

1 15-ounce can pumpkin puree

¼ cup honey

¼ cup blackstrap molasses

2 large eggs

1 teaspoon pure vanilla extract

1 teaspoon baking soda

2 teaspoons ground cinnamon

1 teaspoon ground ginger

2 teaspoons ground cloves

1 cup raw, unsalted chopped nuts: walnuts, slivered almonds, pecans

1 cup raw, unsalted seeds: sunflower, chia, pumpkin

1 cup hemp seeds

DIRECTIONS

Step 1. Preheat the oven to 350°F.

Step 2. Combine all of the ingredients in a large bowl.

Step 3. Drop 2 tablespoons of dough per cookie onto a lightly oiled baking sheet. Space about 2 inches apart.

Step 4. Bake for 15 minutes.

Swift Tip

- I keep a batch of these in the freezer so I have them on hand for Swift "S'mores." Spread some natural nut butter between two cookies for a satisfying, high-fiber treat.

Three-Berry Almost Pie

Preheat the oven to 350°F. In a small ramekin or baking dish, layer in ½ cup of frozen or fresh mixed berries and toss with ½ teaspoon of chia seeds. Top with a drizzle of maple syrup and cinnamon or nutmeg to taste. Top with flaxseed (ground or whole) and bake for about 15 minutes, or until the fruit is bubbling. Remove from the oven, let stand for 3 minutes until cool and enjoy!

One Food Five Swift Ways!

FRUIT: Strawberry

Smoothie: Add frozen strawberries to perk up a smoothie.

Salad: Toss fresh strawberries on your green salad.

Soup: Complement the flavor of a squash soup with fresh strawberries.

Side: Have a side of strawberries along with your morning eggs.

Snack: A perfect fiber-rich, blood sugar–friendly snack, especially when fresh in season.

VEGETABLE: Kale

Smoothie: Green up your smoothie with a handful of kale.

Salad: Massage some kale leaves with extra-virgin olive oil, then add some lemon juice and other veggies for a kalicious salad!

Soup: Chop up kale and add to any of your favorite soup recipes.

Side: Steam up some kale and then drizzle with olive oil and a splash of lemon juice.

Snack: Make your own kale chips.

WHOLE GRAIN: Quinoa

Smoothie: Toss some cooked quinoa into a smoothie for a nutrient and flavor boost!

Salad: Use as a base for a hearty salad.

Soup: Substitute quinoa for pasta in any of your favorite soup recipes.

Side: A quick-cooking side to complement any entrée.

Snack: Explore sprouted quinoa snacks by Perfect Snaque!

LEGUME (PLANT PROTEIN): Chickpea

Smoothie: Add a spoonful of hummus for protein and creaminess.

Salad: Toss some chickpeas in a salad for a protein hit.

Soup: Add some chickpeas to a veggie soup or salad for a protein perk.

Side: Season up your cooked (canned is OK) chickpeas with your favorite spice blend.

Snack: Spice up some chickpeas; drain, toss with olive oil and an herbal blend and bake at 350°F for 1 hour; a crunchy grab-and-go snack.

ANIMAL PROTEIN: Egg

Smoothie: Add a hard-boiled egg to a smoothie for a protein boost.

Salad: Slice up a hard-boiled egg on a salad.

Soup: Try egg drop soup in a miso broth.

Side: A curry egg salad is a delicious side to a veg-loaded meal.

Snack: Hard-boiled egg for the road.

FERMENTED DAIRY: Yogurt

Smoothie: Cream up your smoothie with a cup of yogurt.

Salad: Whip up a minted or curried yogurt dressing to top your salad.

Soup: Dollop a spoonful or two of yogurt in your favorite soup.

Side: Cucumber Raita (page 294) is a delicious side to cool the heat from spicy curry.

Snack: The perfect snack when you are in the mood for something creamy and topped with berries, coconut, a sprinkle of unsweetened cocoa powder or your favorite spice!

FAT: Walnuts

Smoothie: Add an omega-3 boost with raw walnuts or a spoonful of walnut butter.

Salad: Sprinkle some raw walnuts to add crunch to your salad.

Soup: Garnish your soup with chopped raw walnuts.

Side: A crunchy addition to any vegetable side dish!

Snack: Toss a few in your purse for a portable snack.

Cucumber Raita

This recipe comes from my friend Caroline Nation and her team of whole food chefs at myfoodmyhealth.com. It's a wonderful online menu and meal planner site and I've been their chief nutrition adviser for years.

Prep Time: 10 minutes
Cook Time: None
Makes: 1 cup

INGREDIENTS

1½ teaspoons cumin seeds (optional)
1 cup plain, unsweetened organic yogurt
¼ medium seedless cucumber, diced small
1 tablespoon chopped fresh mint
Pinch of sea salt and freshly ground black pepper

DIRECTIONS

Step 1. In a small cast-iron skillet, toast the cumin over medium heat, stirring constantly, until the seeds are fragrant, about 1 minute.

Step 2. Transfer the toasted cumin seeds to a spice grinder or use a mortar and pestle and grind into powder.

Step 3. Mix together the yogurt, cucumber, mint, cumin seeds and a pinch of salt and pepper to taste. Serve chilled.

Swift Shopping List

Use this handy shopping list to save time and spare yourself from unhealthy distractions in those supermarket middle aisles. Feel free to adapt this list based on your favorite recipes. And remember, ingredients do matter, so choose the highest-quality food possible!

Pantry

Beans and Legumes (dry and canned)

- ☐ Adzuki
- ☐ Black
- ☐ Cannellini
- ☐ Garbanzo (chickpea)
- ☐ Lentils
- ☐ Mung
- ☐ Pinto
- ☐ Split peas

Canned Goods (BPA-free)

- ☐ Fish (anchovy, skipjack tuna, salmon, sardines)
- ☐ Pumpkin
- ☐ Tomatoes

Chocolate and Sweeteners

- ☐ Blackstrap molasses
- ☐ Cocoa (butter, nibs, powder)
- ☐ Coconut (creamed, flakes, flour, manna)
- ☐ Dark chocolate (at least 70 percent cacao)
- ☐ Honey (raw, local)
- ☐ Maple syrup (100 percent pure)

Dried Fruits (unsweetened, unsulfured)

Condiments and Such

- ☐ Broth
- ☐ Coffee (organic)

- ☐ Dijon mustard
- ☐ Dried herbs and spices
- ☐ Ketchup
- ☐ Marinara sauce
- ☐ Salsa
- ☐ Sea salt
- ☐ Sea vegetables (kombu, arame, dulse, nori)
- ☐ Sun-dried tomatoes
- ☐ Tamari, gluten-free
- ☐ Teas and herbal teas
- ☐ Vinegars (apple cider, balsamic, red wine)

Nuts and Nut Butters (raw, unsalted)

- ☐ Almonds
- ☐ Brazil nuts
- ☐ Cashews
- ☐ Macadamia
- ☐ Peanuts
- ☐ Pecans
- ☐ Walnuts

Oils (cold expeller pressed)

- ☐ Coconut oil
- ☐ Extra-virgin olive oil
- ☐ Grapeseed oil
- ☐ Sesame oil
- ☐ Walnut oil

Seeds and Seed Butters (natural, raw, unsalted)

- ☐ Chia
- ☐ Flax
- ☐ Pumpkin
- ☐ Sesame

- ☐ Sunflower
- ☐ Tahini

Whole Grains (gluten-free)

- ☐ Amaranth
- ☐ Buckwheat (kasha)
- ☐ Millet
- ☐ Quinoa
- ☐ Rice (black, brown, red)
- ☐ Steel-cut oats
- ☐ Teff
- ☐ Wild rice

Refrigerator and Freezer

Fats

- ☐ Butter
- ☐ Ghee

Fermented/Cultured Foods

- ☐ Kefir
- ☐ Kimchi
- ☐ Miso
- ☐ Pickles
- ☐ Sauerkraut
- ☐ Vegetables
- ☐ Yogurt (plain, unsweetened)

Frozen

- ☐ Fish
- ☐ Fruits
- ☐ Vegetables
- ☐ Vegetarian burgers

Nondairy Beverages (unsweetened)

☐ Almond

☐ Coconut

☐ Hemp seed

☐ Rice

☐ Soy

Produce (choose what's fresh, local and in season!)

☐ Fresh herbs and spices

☐ Fruits

☐ Leafy greens

☐ Roots and tubers

☐ Vegetables

Protein

☐ Beef

☐ Cheese

☐ Chicken

☐ Eggs

☐ Fish

☐ Tempeh

☐ Tofu

☐ Turkey

---

*For recommendations on brands, visit http://www.kathieswift.com.

ACKNOWLEDGMENTS

This book has been the collaborative effort of a dedicated team of individuals who believe in me and in the message of *The Swift Diet*:

Joe Hooper, friend, coauthor and gifted journalist, recognized and valued my work of many years and was eager to shape my thoughts and teachings through countless hours of animated conversation and interviews. We share a love of science, a quest for knowledge and a desire to make it meaningful. Not only am I deeply grateful to work with such a skilled writer, but in the midst of grueling deadlines, Joe was always kind and steadfast in the deliverables.

My husband, Dan, lifelong friend and trusted copilot at the computer and in the kitchen, has more checklists and spreadsheets than anyone can imagine.

My beautiful daughter, Kadan, loving mother, accomplished attorney and inventive home cook, created and tested many of the recipes in this book, borne out of her love of food and health.

My inspiring son, Michael, global adventurist and thinker, who always asked the right questions that led me to a deeper examination of the book in progress.

Kate Doyle Hooper, writer and culinarian, added her wit and creativity to Chapter 7, "The 4-week Swift Plan," and her organizational skills to Chapter 8, "Recipes," making it a more delicious read.

With a stroke of her ingenious pen, our artist, Donna Mehalko, made the illustrations reflect the heart of the manuscript and the beauty of women.

Irina Lisker, MD, consummate healthy living advocate, lent her capable touch to the Swift Plan chapter and ardently pushed me to the finish line.

Amy Jarck, friend, steadfast assistant and recipe analyst, always guides me with her wisdom and thoughtfulness.

I am grateful to my team of accomplished integrative dietitians and culinary nutritionists for their unique contributions: Mary Beth Augustine, dietary supplement content adviser; Sarah Clark, nutrition fact-checker extraordinaire; Monique Richards, healing foods enthusiast; Stefanie Sacks, impassioned food activist and talented chef and Alicia Trocker, whose encouragement was never ending. As well, U.C. Davis microbiologist Maria Marco expanded my fermented food horizons.

Reba Schecter and Jennifer Young lent their expertise to Chapter 6 (Reba on exercise, Jenne on yoga). Whether it's on the yoga mat or the bike path, Rollerblading, ice skating, qigong-ing or hiking in the Berkshires woods, you inspire me to move with joy!

Our determined agent, Linda Loewenthal, trusted the message of *The Swift Diet* and the nutritional and literary chemistry of Joe and me.

The team at Penguin/Hudson Street Press, led by our mindful and keen editor, Caroline Sutton, and including Brittney Ross, Ashley Pattison, Kathryn Santora, Courtney Nobile, Katie Hurley, Norina Frabotta, Susan Schwartz, Daniel Lagin and Jaya Miceli, invested time, energy and heart into the success of this book.

I would like to thank Dr. Mark Hyman, functional medicine leader and friend, who continues to amaze me with his passion to change the American food system to improve the health of our nation, now and for future generations.

Thank you to my mentors and colleagues at three institutions in the integrative health care mecca of the Berkshires: Canyon Ranch, Kripalu Center for Yoga and Health and the UltraWellness Center.

Thank you to my clients and students who have taught me so much over the years through your stories, your struggles and your successes.

And, finally, thank you to the reader, willing, and I hope eager, to embark on this journey with me!

FAQS

Q: What happens if I follow the Swift Plan and the weight stops coming off before I hit my weight-loss goals?

A: The first thing to do is to take a close look at how and what you're eating. Are you eating with awareness, slowly, mindfully? Or are you speed-eating? Are the MicroMenders taking a backseat in your kitchen to the MicroMenaces; for instance, those processed foods with their crowded labels of ingredients? Have you been less than diligent about avoiding foods that you have an adverse reaction to? Keep in mind that beverages can be a sneaky source of calories. Are you drinking your calories in the form of sweetened teas or lattes? Are you using wine to unwind after a long day? Poor food and drink choices can drive weight gain (or slow weight loss) via systemic inflammation.

When you're satisfied that your diet is on track, then it's time to take a deep, relaxing breath. You're at the weight your body wants to be, taking into account your lifestyle at this moment—the stress you're under, the amount of sleep and exercise you get. This is a plateau, or what I like to call a "holding pattern," your body's time to "just be." Trust in yourself and in your plan. This can be a moment of grace, where real self-knowledge begins. Assess the totality of your life. Maybe you can spend an extra half hour on the bike path or at the gym to push up your daily calorie burn.

Maybe you can reorganize your schedule to get an extra hour of sleep at night—remember that sleep deprivation can pump up stress hormones that in turn drive up insulin levels, getting in the way of weight loss. And remember that the trade-off—more gym time, for instance—isn't *necessarily* worth it. Maybe it would cut into valuable family time. It's your decision. Follow your "gut" feelings. And don't be mesmerized by a number on a scale. *How do you feel?* More energetic? If you aren't feeling better, talk with your health care provider, and perhaps some testing, including a thyroid or iron profile, would be in order.

How do you look? Do your clothes feel better on you? Let the body composition tests on page 188 in Chapter 6 be your guide to healthy weight. Allow your body time to recalibrate. Allow yourself time to recharge your batteries and refresh your spirit by embracing the healing mantra of *whole foods, whole person, whole life.*

Q: What happens if I follow the Swift Plan and at the end of four weeks, my digestive symptoms haven't improved much or at all?

A: Perhaps you're not being as scrupulous as you need to be about avoiding a particular food or food ingredient. Maybe it's one or more of the other FODMAP potential irritants that are causing the problem. You'll want to follow the elimination guidelines that I introduced on page 90 in Chapter 3, and in more detail on page 215 in Chapter 7, eliminating one food at a time and observing your body's reaction.

Once you're confident you're doing everything you can with diet, the next step is—give it more time! Digestive issues can respond to dietary changes in a few days, or a few months! After the four weeks of the Swift Plan, stay the careful eating course for another four to six weeks to see if you notice improvement. And keep in mind, we're talking here about intermittent, annoying but not incapacitating digestive problems. Acute or chronic symptoms should send you to your doctor. But even for less severe lingering problems, consider seeking out the counsel of a nutritionist who can use the Swift Diet as a foundation to help you unmask other potential dietary problems and tailor your eating plan accordingly.

If the digestive upset goes much beyond two months, then it is time to search out a health care provider. The problem could be microscopic—you may want to consider medical tests to identify and treat unwelcome guests such as nasty bacterial strains, fungi and parasites. Identifying the root causes is important. One of my favorite MDs in the field is Dr. Robynne Chutkan, gastroenterologist and founder of the Digestive Center for Women in Washington, DC, who takes a holistic approach.

Q: I love the recipes in the Swift Diet. But do I have to give up some of my favorite foods and recipes? There's no Swift dish that closely resembles them.

A: Not at all! You can take any recipe, as long as the ingredients are mostly healthy, whole foods, and "Swift-ize" them by following the proportions of the Swift Plate on page 95 in Chapter 4. Is the recipe you're following built around veggies? Is the protein lean and clean? Do you have any herbs or spices in it? If it includes a starch or grain, is it a whole food choice (butternut squash, quinoa, potato) instead of a highly processed edible? Are the oils or fats in your recipe high quality? When you've really internalized the recipes in Chapter 8, you'll be able to send your own personal favorites through "recipe rehab." For instance, your old fried chicken dish might become something like my Pecan-Crusted Chicken with Swiss Chard and Orange-Scented Carrots (page 263). Or instead of the usual mac 'n' cheese, use a bean pasta and a creamy whipped tofu sauce with a high-quality cheese and spices for added flavor. You'll get plenty of ideas beyond the recipes I've provided by searching out the cookbooks that I've included in my Suggested Reading list (page 319).

Q: I'm not a recipe follower. I want to whip up quick, healthy meals with the ingredients I have in my kitchen. How do I get started?

A: I've got a handy "real foods" menu template for you. And refer to the Swift Shopping List on p. 295, and the lists of healthy foods in Chapter 4, for creative possibilities. Check out the Finding "High" FODMAPs list on

p. 81 to see if there are any foods that you're better off avoiding for now. And remember to stay tuned in to your physical hunger. Follow or adapt the suggested portions below to meet your needs.

Swift Real Foods Sample Menu

Breakfast

Protein: 2 eggs *or* 2 ounces wild lox *or* 4 ounces scrambled seasoned tofu

Non-Starchy Vegetables: 2 cups steamed greens (spinach, for example) *or* other non-starchy vegetables

Fruit: 1 cup berries *or* 1 medium-size piece of fresh fruit *or* 2 small pieces of fruit (kiwi, for example)

Fat: 2 tablespoons nuts or seeds *or* 1 tablespoon natural nut butter

Lunch

Protein: 1 cup cooked (or canned) beans/lentils *or* 3 ounces baked chicken or turkey (about the size of a deck of cards)

Non-Starchy Vegetables: Build a healthy salad with at least 3 cups non-starchy vegetables (for example, leafy greens, cucumber, tomatoes, etc.) and 2 tablespoons of fermented veggies such as ginger carrots

Starchy Vegetable or Gluten-Free Whole Grain: 1 cup starchy vegetable *or* ½ cup cooked gluten-free grain such as quinoa

Fruit: 1 cup berries *or* 1 medium-size piece of fresh fruit *or* 2 small pieces of fruit

Fat: ½ tablespoon extra-virgin olive oil (to be used as a dressing with fresh lemon or lime wedges and herbs) and 2 tablespoons avocado

Dinner

Protein: 3 ounces grilled fish (about the size of a deck of cards) *or* 4 ounces tempeh

Non-Starchy Vegetables: at least 2 cups steamed vegetables and raw salad (if desired)

Starchy Vegetable or Gluten-Free Whole Grain: 1 cup starchy vegetable (sweet potato, for example) *or* ½ cup cooked gluten-free grain (wild rice, for example)

Fat: 1 tablespoon herb pesto and ½ tablespoon extra-virgin olive oil (to be used as a dressing with fresh lemon or lime wedges and herbs)

Snack(s) (if physically hungry): Choose an item from the snack list on page 285 (for example, 1 cup plain, unsweetened yogurt with coconut and a dash of allspice).

Q: My job requires a lot of business dinners, especially when I travel for work. How can I possibly stay on track with my program when I'm eating out so much?

A: It's true, you don't have the same level of control when someone else is doing the cooking, but here are some tips that can definitely help minimize the fallout from eating out.

1. Destination: Whenever possible, have some say in the choice of the restaurant and preview the menu online to see what items will be compatible with your needs, or which ones can be easily adapted to suit them.
2. Don't go hungry: Before you head out, curb your appetite with at least 12 ounces of water plus a light, healthy snack. A piece of fruit or table-spoon of nut butter should do the trick. And once you're at the restau-rant table, trade the bread basket for a dish of olives. Bread is a trap,

there to keep you busy until dinner arrives. Don't fall for it. Banish the bread and munch on olives or crudités instead.

3. Beverages: Ask for water as soon as you're seated. When the server asks for drink orders, skip the pre-meal cocktails and order sparkling water, unsweetened ice tea or water with bitters instead. If you do decide to enjoy a glass of wine or a cocktail, order it with your meal and sip slowly.

4. Ask and don't receive: Tell your server you can't eat certain things: gluten, flour, dairy-based items. These days, most restaurants train their staff to be knowledgeable about the ingredients in the food they serve.

5. Double the veggies and keep it simple: The more veggies the better, so make yours a double, and hold the butter or sauces. Order your fish, shellfish, poultry or meat naked, as in unbreaded, un-sauced and simply prepared with herbs and spices.

6. Olive oil and lemon, and hold the dressing: Ask for dressing on the side and request a side of extra-virgin olive oil and fresh lemon or lime wedges so you, not the sous chef, are in charge of dressing your veggies and salad.

7. Dine with awareness: Remember, dining out is a social event, so enjoy and savor the occasion, not just the meal. Eat slowly, breathe slowly and rest your fork between bites. No need to rush.

8. Embrace the doggie bag: So many restaurant meals are enormous, but you don't have to clean your plate! Instead, when the meal arrives, discreetly split the meal in two and ask for a takeout container, so you can enjoy the leftovers the next day.

9. Drink your dessert: Trade the post-dinner tiramisu for a cup of soothing mint tea or a decaf cappuccino with a dash of cinnamon. If a tempting dessert is an absolute must, then order it with extra forks so everyone at the table gets a bite.

Q: What happens if I fall off the wagon and go back to my old eating habits? What then?

A: Relapses, big and small, happen to all of us. Of course, you want to recommit to the Swift Diet program. But this is the time to learn something from the relapse that you can use moving forward. Make a list of the food triggers that contributed to wandering off course and come up with some strategies to disarm them. Here's an excellent all-purpose "3-D" strategy. You crave a sweet or fatty food that you know is within easy reach. (Ideally, your kitchen and pantry are *not* the sources of these diet-busters—they've been "rehabbed" at the beginning of the Swift Plan.) The first D is "delay": give yourself five minutes before you eat the food. Often, the craving will go away before you get to the rest of the D's! If not, the second D is "distract." Do something soothing or engaging to take your mind off the food. Have a list of quick, easy go-to activities: call a friend, go outdoors, clean a closet, play with a pet, knit. The third D is "decide." Check in with your hunger. Is it really physical or is it more emotional or stress related? Is it born out of habit? If you decide that your hunger is physical, acknowledge it, honor it and then make a conscious food decision. Maybe a piece of fruit would satisfy the hunger just as well—better, really—than the cookie.

You know what? Most often a relapse isn't about food. It's about life. These challenges really are our opportunity to examine what, in the largest sense, is nourishing us and what is depleting us. "Digesting your life," as I like to say. Go back to the mindful and mind-body practices I introduced you to in Chapter 2 and Chapter 6. They can be a wonderful way to bring awareness to what's going on in your life. They can help you detach from the anxieties that can distract you from what's important, not just in your eating plan, but in every aspect of your life.

NOTES

Chapter 1

5 **a major factor driving the rise of obesity:** Blaser MJ and Falkow S (2009). "What are the consequences of the disappearing human microbiome." *Nature Reviews Microbiology* 7(12):887–94. doi:10.1038/nrmicro2245.

6 **In a landmark 2013 study:** Le Chatelier E, Nielsen T, Qin J, et al. (2013). "Richness of human gut microbiome correlates with metabolic markers." *Nature* 500(7464):541–46. doi:10.1038/nature12506.

6 **49 subjects who were overweight were put on a lower-calorie:** Cotillard A, Kennedy SP, Kong LC, et al. (2013). "Dietary intervention impact on gut microbial gene richness." *Nature* 500(7464):585–88. doi:10.1038/nature12480.

7 **150 overweight men and women on a diet:** Sanchez M, Darimont C, Drapeau V, et al. (2013). "Effect of Lactobacillus rhamnosus CGMCC1.3724 supplementation on weight loss and maintenance in obese men and women." *British Journal of Nutrition* 3:1–13.

9 **gut microbiome changed dramatically:** David LA, Maurice CF, Carmody RN, et al. (2014). "Diet rapidly and reproducibly alters the human gut microbiome." *Nature* 505(7484):559–63. doi:10.1038/nature12820.

10 **that sends the brain a similar fullness message:** Frost G, Sleeth ML, Sahuri-Arisoylu M, et al. (2014). "The short-chain fatty acid acetate reduces appetite via a central homeostatic mechanism." *Nature Communications* 5:3611. doi:10.1038/ncomms4611.

24 **develop autoimmune diseases or allergies:** Abrahamsson TR, Jakobsson HE, Andersson AF, et al. (2013). "Low gut microbiota in early infancy precedes asthma at school age." *Clinical and Experimental Allergy.* doi:10.1111/cea.12253.

24 **less diversity in the macro world leads to:** Haahtela T, Holgate S, Pawankar R,

et al. (2013). "WAO Special Committee on Climate Change and Biodiversity. The biodiversity hypothesis and allergic disease: world allergy organization position statement." *World Allergy Organization Journal* 6(1):1–18. doi:10.1186/1939-4551-6-3.

Chapter 2

29 **guilty eaters had gained more weight:** Kuijer RG, Boyce JA (2014). "Chocolate cake. Guilt or celebration? Associations with healthy eating attitudes, perceived behavioural control, intentions and weight-loss." *Appetite* 74:48–54. doi:10.1016/j.appet.2013.11.013.

29 **questionnaires given to over five thousand:** Scherwitz L, Kesten D (2005). "Seven eating styles linked to overeating, overweight, and obesity." *Explore* (NY) 1(5):342–59.

38 **when we *don't* eat, the body takes advantage:** Takahashi T (2012). "Mechanism of interdigestive migrating motor complex." *Journal of Neurogastroenterology* 18(3): 246–57. doi:10.5056/jnm.2012.18.3.246.

40 **group of gregarious mice into a group of timid:** Desbonnet L, Garrett L, Clarke G, et al. (2010). "Effects of the probiotic *Bifidobacterium infantis* in the maternal separation model of depression." *Neuroscience* 170(4):1179–88. doi:10.1016/j.

40 **gut bacteria were "influencing":** Collins SM, Surette M, Bercik P (2012). "The interplay between the intestinal microbiota and the brain." *Nature Reviews: Microbiology* 10(11):735–42. doi:10.1038/nrmicro2876.

40 **probiotic strains altered the rodents' production:** Selhub EM, Logan AC, Bested AC (2014). "Fermented foods, microbiota, and mental health: ancient practice meets nutritional psychiatry." *Journal of Physiological Anthropology* 33:2. doi:10.1186/1880-6805-33-2.

40 **women who ate the yogurt saw changes:** Tillisch K, Labus J, Kilpatrick L, et al. (2013). "Consumption of fermented milk product with probiotic modulates brain activity." *Gastroenterology* 144(7):1394–401, 1401.e1-4. doi:10.1053/j.gastro.2013.02.043.

45 **counterparts who received no training:** Daubenmier J, Kristeller J, Hecht FM, et al. (2011). "Mindfulness intervention for stress eating to reduce cortisol and abdominal fat among overweight and obese women: an exploratory randomized controlled study." *Journal of Obesity* 2011:1–13. doi:10.1155/2011/651936.

Chapter 3

52 **in the form of seeds and plants and fruits:** Spreadbury I (2012). "Comparison with ancestral diets suggests dense acellular carbohydrates promote an inflammatory microbiota, and may be the primary dietary cause of leptin resistance and obesity." *Diabetes, Metabolic Syndrome and Obesity: Targets and Therapy* 5:175–89. doi:10.2147/DMSO.S33473.

53 **high levels of consumption:** Mozaffarian D, Hao T, Rimm EB, et al. (2011).

"Changes in diet and lifestyle and long-term weight gain in women and men." *New England Journal of Medicine* 364(25):2392–404. doi:10.1056/NEJMoa1014296.

55 **substituting one serving of beans:** Mattei J, Hu FB, Campos H (2011). "A higher ratio of beans to white rice is associated with lower cardiometabolic risk factors in Costa Rican adults." *American Journal of Clinical Nutrition* 94(3):869–76. doi:10.3945/ajcn.111.013219.

55 **my friend Dr. David Ludwig:** Ebbeling CB, Swain JF, Feldman HA, et al. (2012). "Effects of dietary composition on energy expenditure during weight-loss maintenance." *Journal of the American Medical Association* 307(24):2627–34. doi:10.1001/jama.2012.6607.

56 **One leading microbiome researcher:** Marcobal A, Southwick AM, Earle KA, et al. (2013). "A refined palate: bacterial consumption of host glycans in the gut." *Glycobiology* 23(9):1038–46. doi: 10.1093/glycob/cwt040.

57 **linked the rich diversity of gut:** Ou J, Carbonero F, Zoetendal EG, et al. (2013). "Diet, microbiota, and microbial metabolites in colon cancer risk in rural Africans and African Americans." *American Journal of Clinical Nutrition* 98(1):111–20. doi:10.3945/ajcn.112.056689.

57 **a foundation of vegetables and fruit:** Konner M, Eaton SB (2010). "Paleolithic nutrition: twenty-five years later." *Nutrition in Clinical Practice* 25: 594. doi:10.1177/088453610385702.

59 **morsel of processed food in this country:** United States Department of Agriculture (2013). "Sugar and sweeteners outlook, NAFTA and world sugar June 2013." Economic Research Service.

60 **regulate sugar the same way:** Lustig RH, Schmidt LA, Brindis CD (2012). "Public health: the toxic truth about sugar." *Nature* 482(7383):27–29. doi:10.1038/482027a.

61 **physiological reasons why people:** Lennerz BS, Alsop DC, Holsen LM, et al. (2013). "Effects of dietary glycemic index on brain regions related to reward and craving in men." *American Journal of Clinical Nutrition* 98(3):641–7. doi:10.3945/ajcn.113.064113.

62 **subjects who consumed the HFCS:** Stanhope KL, Schwarz JM, Keim NL, et al. (2009). "Consuming fructose-sweetened, not glucose-sweetened, beverages increases visceral adiposity and lipids and decreases insulin sensitivity in overweight/obese humans." *Journal of Clinical Investigation* 119(5):1322–34. doi:10.1172/JCI37385.

62 **confusing our hunger signals:** Sievenpiper JL, de Souza RJ, Mirrahimi A, et al. (2012). "Effect of fructose on body weight in controlled feeding trials: a systematic review and meta-analysis." *Annals of Internal Medicine* 156(4):291–304. doi:10.7326/0003-4819-156-4-201202210-00007.

63 **overweight and obese was skyrocketing:** Mozaffarian D, Appel LJ, Van Horn L (2011). "Components of a cardioprotective diet: new insights." *Circulation* 123(24): 2870–91. doi:10.1161/CIRCULATIONAHA.110.968735.

63 **who took their yogurt with simple table sugar:** Feijó Fde M, Ballard CR, Foletto

KC, et al. (2013). "Saccharin and aspartame, compared with sucrose, induce greater weight gain in adult Wistar rats, at similar total caloric intake levels." *Appetite* 60(1):203–7. doi:10.1016/j.appet.2012.10.009.

64 **helpful bacteria in the gut:** Schiffman SS, Rother KI (2013). "Sucralose, a synthetic organochlorine sweetener: overview of biological issues." *Journal of Toxicology and Environmental Health* 16(7):399–451. doi:10.1080/10937404.2013.842523.

65 **But in microbiome study:** Cani PD, Osto M, Geurts L, et al. (2012). "Involvement of gut microbiota in the development of low-grade inflammation and type 2 diabetes associated with obesity." *Gut Microbes* 3(4):279–88.

65 **dietary fat, especially animal fat:** Kemp DM (2013). "Does chronic low-grade endotoxemia define susceptibility of obese humans to insulin resistance via dietary effects on gut microbiota?" *Adipocyte* 2(3):188–90. doi:10.4161/adip.24776.

66 **people who consume a lot of saturated:** Estadella D, da Penha Oller do Nascimento CM, Oyama LM, et al. (2013). "Lipotoxicity: effects of dietary saturated and trans-fatty acids." *Mediators of Inflammation* 2013:137579. doi:10.1155/2013/137579.

66 **ingestion of 300 calories:** Deopurkar R, Ghanim H, Friedman J, et al. (2010). "Differential effects of cream, glucose, and orange juice on inflammation, endotoxin, and the expression of Toll-like receptor-4 and suppressor of cytokine signaling-3." *Diabetes Care* 33(5):991–97. doi:10.2337/dc09-1630.

66 **through a healthy gut microbiota:** Tuohy KM, Fava F, Viola R (2014). " 'The way to a man's heart is through his gut microbiota'—dietary pro- and prebiotics for the management of cardiovascular risk." *Proceedings of the Nutrition Society* 73(2): 172–85. doi: 10.1017/S0029665113003911.

66 **a lot of the older research has been reexamined:** Chowdhury R, Warnakula S, Kunutsor S, et al. (2014). "Association of dietary, circulating, and supplement fatty acids with coronary risk: a systematic review and meta-analysis." *Annals of Internal Medicine* 160(6): 398–406. doi:10.7326/M13-1788.

67 **omega-6 fatty acids get converted:** Vannice G, Rasmussen H (2014). "Position of the Academy of Nutrition and Dietetics: dietary fatty acids for healthy adults." *Journal of the Academy of Nutrition and Dietetics* 114(1):136–53. doi:10.1016/j .jand.2013.11.001.

68 **Still, scientists have succeeded:** Kim E, Coelho D, Blachier F (2013). "Review of the association between meat consumption and risk of colorectal cancer." *Nutrition Research* 33(12):983–94. doi:10.1016/j.nutres.2013.07.018.

69 **speeding up our own aging process:** Uribarri J, Woodruff S, Goodman S, et al. (2010). "Advanced glycation end products in foods and a practical guide to their reduction in the diet." *Journal of the American Dietetic Association* 110(6):911–16. e12. doi:10.1016/j.jada.2010.03.018.

70 **type 2 diabetes with a vegan:** Fallucca F, Porrata C, Fallucca A, et al (2014). "Influence of diet on gut microbiota, inflammation and type 2 diabetes mellitus. First

experience with macrobiotic Ma-Pi 2 diet." *Diabetes/Metabolism Research and Reviews* 30(Suppl. 1):48–54. doi:10.1002/dmrr.2518.

75 **gluten intolerance may be linked:** Catassi C, Bai JC, Bonaz B, et al. (2013). "Non-Celiac Gluten sensitivity: the new frontier of gluten related disorders." *Nutrients* 5(10):3839–53. doi: 10.3390/nu5103839.

75 **worse odds than the people with celiac disease:** Peters U, Askling J, Gridley G, et al (2003). "Causes of death in patients with celiac disease in a population-based Swedish cohort." *Archives of Internal Medicine* 163(13):1566–72.

79 **produce progressively less lactase:** Brüssow H (2013). "Nutrition, population growth and disease: a short history of lactose." *Environmental Microbiology* 15(8):2154–61. doi:10.1111/1462-2920.12117.

79 **suspect that gluten intolerance often sets:** Campbell AK, Matthews SB, Vassel N, et al. (2010). "Bacterial metabolic 'toxins': a new mechanism for lactose and food intolerance, and irritable bowel syndrome." *Toxicology* 278(3):268–76. doi:10.1016/j.tox.2010.09.001.

80 **Nestlé Research Center in Switzerland:** Brüssow H (2013). "Nutrition, population growth and disease: a short history of lactose." *Environmental Microbiology* 15(8):2154–61. doi:10.1111/1462-2920.12117.

80 **over 70 percent of the subjects lessened:** Shepherd SJ, Gibson PR (2006). "Fructose malabsorption and symptoms of irritable bowel syndrome: guidelines for effective dietary management." *Journal of the American Dietetic Association* 106(10):1631–39.

87 **binge drinking, can increase gut:** Reding KW, Cain KC, Jarrett ME, et al. (2013). "Relationship between patterns of alcohol consumption and gastrointestinal symptoms among patients with irritable bowel syndrome." *Journal of Gastroenterology* 108(2):270–76. doi:10.1038/ajg.2012.414.

88 **in adults as well as children:** Skypala I (2011). "Adverse food reactions—an emerging issue for adults." *Journal of the American Dietetic Association* 111:1877–91. doi:10.1016/j.jada.2011.09.001.

Chapter 4

96 **our leading killer:** Brock JF, Gordon H (1959). "Ischaemic heart disease in African populations." *Postgraduate Medical Journal* 35(402):223–32.

97 **any connection between saturated fat consumption and heart disease:** Chowdhury R, Warnakula S, Kunutsor S, et al. (2014). "Association of dietary, circulating, and supplement fatty acids with coronary risk: a systematic review and meta-analysis." *Annals of Internal Medicine* 160(6): 398–406. doi:10.7326/M13-1788.

97 **fewer heart attacks and less heart disease:** Threapleton DE, Greenwood DC, Evans CE, et al. (2013). "Dietary fibre intake and risk of cardiovascular disease: systematic review and meta-analysis." *British Medical Journal* 347:f6879. doi:10.1136/bmj.f6879.

101 **diet rich in vegetables and fruits . . . tamp down:** Liu RH (2013). "Dietary bioactive compounds and their health implications." *Journal of Food Science* 78 Suppl 1:A18–25. doi:10.1111/1750-3841.12101.

104 **The polyphenols work to stabilize blood:** Hanhineva K, Törrönen R, Bondia-Pons I, et al. (2010). "Impact of dietary polyphenols on carbohydrate metabolism." *International Journal of Molecular Sciences* 11(4):1365–402. doi:10.3390/ijms11041365.

104 **common species of gut bacteria:** Rastmanesh R (2011). "High polyphenol, low probiotic diet for weight loss because of intestinal microbiota interaction." *Chemico-Biological Interactions* 189(1–2):1–8. doi:10.1016/j.cbi.2010.10.002.

104 **for many of those vaunted health benefits:** Tzounis X, Rodriguez-Mateos A, Vulevic J, et al. (2011). "Prebiotic evaluation of cocoa-derived flavanols in healthy humans by using a randomized, controlled, double-blind, crossover intervention study." *American Journal of Clinical Nutrition* 93(1):62–72. doi:10.3945/ajcn.110.000075.

106 **raises the risk of breast cancer:** Fowke JH, Longcope C, Hebert JR (2000). "Brassica vegetable consumption shifts estrogen metabolism in healthy postmenopausal women." *Cancer Epidemiology Biomarkers Prevention* 9(8):773–79.

112 **that fruit consumption:** Ludwig DS (2013). "Examining the health effects of fructose." *Journal of the American Medical Association* 310(1):33–34. doi:10.1001/jama.2013.6562.

113 **the consumption of blueberries increased the number:** Menon R, Watson SE, Thomas LN, et al. (2013). "Diet complexity and estrogen receptor β status affect the composition of the murine intestinal microbiota." *Applied Environmental Microbiology* 79(18):5763–73. doi:10.1128/AEM.01182-13.

113 **may stimulate the growth of the gut's:** Monro JA (2013). "Kiwifruit, carbohydrate availability, and the glycemic response." *Advances in Food Nutrition and Research* 68:257–71. doi:10.1016/B978-0-12-394294-4.00014-6.

117 **folate, which reduces homocysteine:** Johnston C (2009). "Functional foods as modifiers of cardiovascular disease." *American Journal of Lifestyle Medicine* 3(1 Suppl):39S–43S.

117 **bacteria breaking down those plant:** Brighenti F, Benini L, Del Rio D, et al. (2006). "Colonic fermentation of indigestible carbohydrates contributes to the second-meal effect." *American Journal of Clinical Nutrition* 83(4):817–22.

118 **phytate also serves as an antioxidant:** Zajdel A, Wilczok A, Węglarz L, et al. (2013). "Phytic acid inhibits lipid peroxidation in vitro." *BioMed Research International* 2013:147307. doi:10.1155/2013/147307.

118 **fiber in the legumes help break:** Markiewicz LH, Honke J, Haros M, et al. (2013). "Diet shapes the ability of human intestinal microbiota to degrade phytate—in vitro studies." *Journal of Applied Microbiology* 115(1):247–59. doi:10.1111/jam.12204.

121 **may be a potent prebiotic:** Metzler-Zebeli BU, Zijlstra RT, Mosenthin R, et al. (2011). "Dietary calcium phosphate content and oat β-glucan influence gastrointes-

tinal microbiota, butyrate-producing bacteria and butyrate fermentation in weaned pigs." *FEMS Microbiology Ecology* 75(3):402–13. doi:10.1111/j.1574-6941.2010.01017.x.

121 **and possibly anticancer effects:** Meydani M (2009). "Potential health benefits of avenanthramides of oats." *Nutrition Reviews* 67(12):731–35. doi:10.1111/j.1753-4887.2009.00256.x.

128 **risk of heart disease by about a third:** Hu FB, Stampfer MJ (1999). "Nut consumption and coronary heart disease: a review of epidemiologic evidence." *Current Atherosclerosis Reports* 1(3):204–9.

128 **our two most reliable friends in the microbiome:** Liu Z, Lin X, Huang G, et al. (2014). "Prebiotic effects of almonds and almond skins on intestinal microbiota in healthy adult humans." *Anaerobe* 26:1–6. doi:10.1016/j.anaerobe.2013.11.007.

129 **adding half an avocado:** Wien M, Haddad E, Oda K, et al. (2013). "A randomized 3x3 crossover study to evaluate the effect of Hass avocado intake on post-ingestive satiety, glucose and insulin levels, and subsequent energy intake in overweight adults." *Nutrition Journal* 12:155. doi:10.1186/1475-2891-12-155.

130 **eaten turmeric, rosemary, cloves:** Percival SS, Vanden Heuvel JP, Nieves CJ, et al. (2012). "Bioavailability of herbs and spices in humans as determined by ex vivo inflammatory suppression and DNA strand breaks." *Journal of the American College of Nutrition* 31(4):288–94.

131 **temporarily turn up the metabolic:** Mattes RD (2011). "Spices and energy balance." *Physiology and Behavior* 107(4):584–90. doi:10.1016/j.physbeh.2011.10.028.

132 **extract from the fresh leaves:** Doddanna SJ, Patel S, Sundarrao MA (2013). "Antimicrobial activity of plant extracts on *Candida albicans*: an in vitro study." *Indian Journal of Dental Research* 24(4):401–5. doi:10.4103/0970-9290.118358.

133 **found most abundantly in green tea:** Hanhineva K, Törrönen R, Bondia-Pons I, et al. (2010). "Impact of dietary polyphenols on carbohydrate metabolism." *International Journal of Molecular Science* 11(4):1365–402. doi:10.3390/ijms11041365.

134 **consumption of dark chocolate:** Hooper L, Kay C, Abdelhamid A, et al. (2012). "Effects of chocolate, cocoa, and flavan-3-ols on cardiovascular health: a systematic review and meta-analysis of randomized trials." *American Journal of Clinical Nutrition* 95(3):740–51. doi:10.3945/ajcn.111.023457.

134 **topical treatment for burns:** Israili ZH (2013). "Antimicrobial properties of honey." *American Journal of Therapeutics.* doi: 10.1097/MJT.0b013e318293b09b.

134 **An antimicrobial when it's applied:** Al-Waili NS, Salom K, Butler G, et al. (2011). "Honey and microbial infections: a review supporting the use of honey for microbial control." *Journal of Medicinal Food* 14(10):1079–96. doi:10.1089/jmf.2010.0161.

136 **Washington University's Dr. Jeffrey Gordon:** Sonnenburg JL, Chen CT, Gordon JI (2006). "Genomic and metabolic studies of the impact of probiotics on a model gut symbiont and host." *PLoS Biology* 4(12):e413.

136 **microbiota to explain the studies:** O'Connor LM, Lentjes MA, Luben RN, et al.

(2014). "Dietary dairy product intake and incident type 2 diabetes: a prospective study using dietary data from a 7-day food diary." *Diabetologia* 57(5):909–17. doi: 10.1007/s00125-014-3176-1.

136 **kimchi to the diet can reduce:** Choi IH, Noh JS, Han JS, et al. (2013). "Kimchi, a fermented vegetable, improves serum lipid profiles in healthy young adults: randomized clinical trial." *Journal of Medicinal Food* 16(3):223–29. doi:10.1089/ jmf.2012.2563.

136 **fermented foods have shown promise:** Lakritz JR, Poutahidis T, Levkovich T, et al. (2013). "Beneficial bacteria stimulate host immune cells to counteract dietary and genetic predisposition to mammary cancer in mice." *International Journal of Cancer*. doi:10.1002/ijc.28702.

138 **tempeh first made its appearance:** Astuti M, Meliala A, Dalais FS, et al. (2000). "Tempe, a nutritious and healthy food from Indonesia." *Asia Pacific Journal of Clinical Nutrition* 9(4):322–25.

138 **antifungal and antibacterial:** Lopitz-Otsoa F, Rementeria A, Elguezabal N, et al. (2006). "Kefir: a symbiotic yeasts-bacteria community with alleged healthy capabilities." *Phytotherapy Research* 23(2):67–74.

138 **bacterial strains from the beverage:** Chen YP, Hsiao PJ, Hong WS, et al. (2012). "Lactobacillus kefiranofaciens M1 isolated from milk kefir grains ameliorates experimental colitis in vitro and in vivo." *Journal of Dairy Science* 95(1):63–74. doi:10.3168/jds.2011-4696.

Chapter 5

151 **herbal supplements from China and India:** Newmaster SG, Grguric M, Shanmughanandhan D, et al. (2013). "DNA barcoding detects contamination and substitution in North American herbal products." *BMC Medicine* 11:222. doi:10.1186/ 1741-7015-11-222.

152 **the academic researchers who have looked:** Hasani-Ranjbar S, Nayebi N, Larijani B, et al. (2009). "A systematic review of the efficacy and safety of herbal medicines used in the treatment of obesity." *World Journal Gastroenterology* 15(25):3073–85.

152 **dietary supplements and weight management:** Lovejoy JC (2013). "Integrative approaches to obesity treatment." *Integrative Medicine: A Clinician's Journal Integrative Medicine* 12(2):30–36.

155 **may directly influence our food preferences:** Norris V, Molina F, Gewirtz, AT (2013). "Hypothesis: bacteria control host appetites." *Journal of Bacteriology* 195(3):411–16.

157 **Popular Probiotic Products:** this list was adapted from: Vieira AT, Teixeira MM, Martins FS (2013). "The role of probiotics and prebiotics in inducing gut immunity." *Frontiers in Immunology* 4(445):1–12.

Chapter 6

177 **established research linking poor:** Chaput JP (2013). "Sleep patterns, diet quality and energy balance." *Physiology and Behavior* pii: S0031-9384(13)00286-2. doi:10.1016/j.physbeh.2013.09.006.

177 **weight fluctuated by only:** Markwald RR, Melanson EL, Smith MR, et al. (2013). "Impact of insufficient sleep on total daily energy expenditure, food intake, and weight gain." *Proceedings of the National Academy of Science* 110(14):5695–700. doi:10.1073/pnas.1216951110.

178 **disrupting the sleep/wake cycle of mice:** Summa KC, Voigt RM, Forsyth CB, et al. (2013). "Disruption of the circadian clock in mice increases intestinal permeability and promotes alcohol-induced hepatic pathology and inflammation." *PLoS One* 8(6):e67102.

179 **adolescents who had TVs in their bedrooms:** Gilbert-Diamond D, Li Z, Adachi-Mejia AM, et al. (2014). "Association of a television in the bedroom with increased adiposity gain in a nationally representative sample of children and adolescents." *JAMA Pediatrics* doi:10.1001/jamapediatrics.2013.3921.

179 **a good night's sleep at the hormonal level:** Wood B, Rea MS, Plitnick B, et al. (2013). "Light level and duration of exposure determine the impact of self-luminous tablets on melatonin suppression." *Applied Ergonomics* 44(2):237–40. doi:10.1016/j.apergo.2012.07.008.

180 **clocks help regulate a host:** Konturek PC, Brzozowski T, Konturek SJ (2011). "Gut clock: implication of circadian rhythms in the gastrointestinal tract." *Journal of Physiology and Pharmacology* 62(2):139–50.

181 **group experienced a mood lift outdoors:** (2007). "Ecotherapy: the green agenda for mental health." *Mind Week Report.* Available at: http://www.mind.org.uk/media/211252/Ecotherapy_The_green_agenda_for_mental_health_Executive_summary.pdf. Accessed March 16, 2014.

181 **the lower the kids' body mass index:** Bell JF, Wilson JS, Liu GC (2008). "Neighborhood greenness and 2-year changes in body mass index of children and youth." *American Journal of Preventive Medicine* 35(6):547–53. doi:10.1016/j.amepre.2008.07.006.

182 **exercise to be as good as or better than:** Naci H, Ioannidis JP (2013). "Comparative effectiveness of exercise and drug interventions on mortality outcomes: metaepidemiological study." *BMJ* 347:f5577. doi:10.1136/bmj.f5577.

188 **a better predictor of heart health:** Gupta S, Kapoor S (2014). "Body adiposity index: its relevance and validity in assessing body fatness of adults." *ISRN Obesity* 2014:243294. doi:10.1155/2014/243294.

194 **overweight in their forties:** Kristal AR, Littman AJ, Benitez D, et al. (2005). "Yoga practice is associated with attenuated weight gain in healthy, middle-aged men and women." *Alternative Therapies in Health and Medicine* 11(4):28–33.

195 **feel more connected to their bodies:** McIver S, McGartland M, O'Halloran P (2009). "'Overeating is not about the food': women describe their experience of a yoga treatment program for binge eating." *Qualitative Health Research* 19(9):1234–45. doi:10.1177/1049732309343954.

195 **yoga was found to be more effective:** Taneja I, Deepak KK, Poojary G, et al. (2004). "Yogic versus conventional treatment in diarrhea-predominant irritable bowel syndrome: a randomized control study." *Applied Psychophysiology and Biofeedback* 29(1):19–33.

201 **improved their blood sugar levels:** Liu X, Miller YD, Burton NW, et al. (2011). "Qigong mind-body therapy and diabetes control. A randomized controlled trial." *American Journal of Preventive Medicine* 41(2):152–58. doi:10.1016/j.amepre .2011.04.007.

SWIFT RESOURCES: BOOKS, DVDS, FILMS, WEB SITES

Suggested Reading

There is a library's worth of good books on food and health, and on living skillfully to heighten your experience of both. Here are some of my favorites that, one way or another, informed and inspired the writing of *The Swift Diet*.

Linda Bacon, PhD. *Health at Every Size: The Surprising Truth About Your Weight*. BenBella Books, 2010.

Jeffrey S. Bland, PhD. *The Disease Delusion: Conquering the Causes of Chronic Illness for a Healthier, Longer, and Happier Life*. Harper Wave, 2014.

Martin J. Blaser, MD. *Missing Microbes: How the Overuse of Antibiotics Is Fueling Our Modern Plagues*. Henry Holt and Co., 2014.

Susan Blum, MD, MPH. *The Immune System Recovery Plan: A Doctor's 4-Step Program to Treat Autoimmune Disease*. Scribner, 2013.

Dan Buettner. *The Blue Zones: Lessons for Living Longer from the People Who've Lived the Longest*. National Geographic, 2010.

Robynne Chutkan, MD. *Gutbliss: A 10-Day Plan to Ban Bloat, Flush Toxins, and Dump Your Digestive Baggage*. Avery, 2013.

Stephen Cope. *The Wisdom of Yoga: A Seeker's Guide to Extraordinary Living*. Bantam, 2007.

Marc David. *The Slow Down Diet: Eating for Pleasure, Energy, and Weight Loss*. Healing Arts Press, 2005.

Brenda Davis, RD, and Vesanto Melina, MS, RD. *Becoming Vegan*, Express Edition. Book Pub Co., 2013.

William Davis, MD. *Wheat Belly*. Rodale Books, 2011.

Danna Faulds. *Go In and In: Poems from the Heart of Yoga.* Peaceable Kingdom Books, 2002.

Michael D. Gershon, MD. *The Second Brain: A Groundbreaking New Understanding of Nervous Disorders of the Stomach and Intestine.* Harper Perennial, 1999.

James S. Gordon, MD. *Unstuck: Your Guide to the Seven-Stage Journey Out of Depression.* Penguin Books, 2009.

Thich Nhat Hanh and Dr. Lilian Cheung. *Savor: Mindful Eating, Mindful Life.* Harper-One. 2011.

Arianna Huffington. *Thrive: The Third Metric to Redefining Success and Creating a Life of Well-Being, Wisdom, and Wonder.* Harmony, 2014.

Mark Hyman, MD. *The Blood Sugar Solution 10-Day Detox.* Little, Brown and Company, 2014.

———. *The UltraMind Solution: Fix Your Broken Brain by Healing Your Body First.* Scribner 2008.

———. *UltraMetabolism: The Simple Plan for Automatic Weight Loss.* Atria Books, 2008.

Alejandro Junger, MD. *Clean Gut: The Breakthrough Plan for Eliminating the Root Cause of Disease and Revolutionizing Your Health.* HarperOne, 2013.

David Katz, MD, and Stacey Colino. *Disease-Proof: The Remarkable Truth About What Makes Us Well.* Hudson Street Press, 2013.

Sandor Ellix Katz. *The Art of Fermentation.* Chelsea Green Publishing, 2012.

Annie B. Kay, MS, RD, RYT. *Every Bite Is Divine.* Life Arts Press, 2007.

David A. Kessler, MD. *The End of Overeating: Taking Control of the Insatiable American Appetite.* Rodale Books, 2010.

William Kotzwinkle, Glenn Murray and Audrey Colman. *Walter, the Farting Dog.* Frog Children's Books, 2001.

Chris Kresser. *Your Personal Paleo Code: The 3-Step Plan to Lose Weight, Reverse Disease, and Stay Fit and Healthy for Life.* Little, Brown and Co., 2013.

Jeff D. Leach. *Honor Thy Symbionts.* CreateSpace Independent Publishing Platform, 2012.

Frank Lipman, MD, and Mollie Doyle. *Revive: Stop Feeling Spent and Start Living Again.* Pocket Books, 2011.

Mark Liponis, MD. *The Hunter/Diet Solution.* Hay House, 2012.

Elizabeth Lipski. *Digestive Wellness: Strengthen the Immune System and Prevent Disease Through Healthy Digestion.* McGraw-Hill, 2011.

Richard Louv. *The Nature Principle: Reconnecting with Life in a Virtual Age.* Algonquin, 2012.

Tieraona Low Dog, MD. *Life Is Your Best Medicine: A Woman's Guide to Health, Healing and Wholeness at Every Age.* National Geographic, 2012.

Robert H. Lustig, MD. *Fat Chance: Beating the Odds Against Sugar, Processed Food, Obesity, and Disease.* Plume, 2013.

Woodson Merrell, MD, with Mary Beth Augustine, MS, RDN, and Hillari Dowdle, RYT. *The Detox Prescription*. Rodale, 2013.

Daphne Miller, MD. *Farmacology: What Innovative Family Farming Can Teach Us About Health and Healing*. William Morrow, 2013.

Michael Moss. *Salt Sugar Fat: How the Food Giants Cooked Us*. Random House Trade Paperbacks, 2014.

Gerard E. Mullin, MD, and Kathie Madonna Swift, MS, RD, LDN. *The Inside Tract: Your Good Gut Guide to Great Digestive Health*. Rodale Books, 2011.

David Perlmutter, MD. *Grain Brain*. Little, Brown and Co., 2013.

Michael Pollan, *Cooked: A Natural History of Transformation*. Penguin Books, 2014.

———. *In Defense of Food*. Penguin Books, 2009.

Mary Roach. *Gulp: Adventures on the Alimentary Canal*. W. W. Norton & Company, 2014.

Jo Robinson. *Eating on the Wild Side*. Little, Brown and Company, 2013.

Aviva Rom, MD. *Botanical Medicine for Women's Health*. Churchill Livingstone, 2009.

Joshua Rosenthal. *Integrative Nutrition: Feed Your Hunger for Health and Happiness*. Integrative Nutrition Publishing, 2014.

Stefanie Sacks, MS, CNS, CDN. *What the Fork (Are You Eating): An Action Plan for Your Pantry and Plate*. Tarcher/Penguin, forthcoming 2014/early 2015.

Diane Sanfilippo. *Practical Paleo: A Customized Approach to Health and a Whole-Foods Lifestyle*. Victory Belt Publishing, 2012.

Mary Shomon. *The Thyroid Diet Revolution: Manage Your Master Gland of Metabolism for Lasting Weight Loss*. William Morrow Paperbacks, 2012.

Liz Vaccariello with Kate Scarlata, RD. *20-Day Tummy: The Revolutionary Diet That Soothes and Shrinks Any Belly Fast*. Readers Digest, 2013.

J. J. Virgin, PhD, CNS. *The Virgin Diet: Drop 7 Foods, Lose 7 Pounds, Just 7 Days*. Harlequin, 2012.

Cookbooks

Leslie Cerier. *Gluten-Free Recipes for the Conscious Cook: A Seasonal Vegetarian Cookbook*. New Harbinger Publications, 2010.

Mark Hyman, MD. *The UltraMetabolism Cookbook: 200 Delicious Recipes That Will Turn on Your Fat-Burning DNA*. Scribner, 2007.

Rebecca Katz with Mat Edelson. *The Longevity Kitchen: Satisfying, Big-Flavor Recipes Featuring the Top 16 Age-Busting Power Foods*. Ten Speed Press, 2013.

Drew Ramsey, MD, and Jennifer Iserloh. *50 Shades of Kale: Fifty Fresh and Satisfying Recipes That Are Bound to Please*. Harper Wave, 2013.

Alissa Segersten and Tom Malterre, MS, CN. *Nourishing Meals: Healthy Gluten-Free Meals for the Whole Family*. Whole Life Press, 2012.

Editors of *Martha Stewart Living. Clean Slate: A Cookbook and Guide: Reset Your Health, Boost Your Energy, and Feel Your Best.* Clarkson Potter, 2014.

Scott Uehlein and Canyon Ranch. *Canyon Ranch: Nourish: Indulgently Healthy Cuisine.* Studio, 2009.

Andrew Weil and Sam Fox with Michael Stebner. *True Food: Seasonable, Sustainable, Simple, Pure.* Little, Brown and Company, 2014.

Editors of *Whole Living* magazine. *Power Foods.* Clarkson Potter, 2010.

DVDs

Dr. Yang Yang's Evidence-based Taiji and Qigong Program: Nurturing Mind, Body, Spirit. www.centerfortaiji.com.

Belleruth Naparstek "guided imagery" DVDs, especially on IBS, irritable bowel disease and sleep, www.healthjourneys.com.

Films/Documentaries

Fed Up: http://fedupmovie.com

"Food": http://articles.mercola.com/sites/articles/archive/2014/01/11/food-documentary.aspx

Food Inc.: www.takepart.com/foodinc

Food Matters: www.foodmatters.TV/food-matters-film

Forks over Knives: www.forksoverknives.com

Web Sites

American College of Gastroenterology
www.gi.org

American Gut Project
http://humanfoodproject.com/americangut

Animal Welfare Approved
www. animalwelfareapproved.org

Body Adiposity Index online calculator (BAI is a new measure of body fat.)
http://easycalculation.com/health/body-adiposity-index.php

Canyon Ranch Health Resort
www.canyonranch.com

Celiac Central
www.celiaccentral.org/

Celiac.com
www.celiac.com/

Center for Food Safety
http://centerforfoodsafety.org/

The Center for Mind-Body Medicine
www.cmbm.org

Center for Science in the Public Interest
http://cspinet.org/index.html

The Centers for Disease Control's online calculator to figure out your optimal vegetable and fruit consumption, based on age, sex and physical activity
http://www.cdc.gov/nutrition/everyone/fruitsvegetables/howmany.html

ConsumerLab.com (for unbiased reviews of natural products/supplements)
www.consumerlab.com

Cultures for Health (to get starter kefir "grains" to make kefir at home)
www.culturesforhealth.com

Dietitians in Integrative and Functional Medicine, a dietetic practice group of the Academy of Nutrition and Dietetics
www.IntegrativeRD.org

Eat Wild: Getting Wild Nutrition from Modern Food
www.eatwild.com/

Environmental Working Group
www.ewg.org

Environmental Working Group's Dirty Dozen/Clean Fifteen list of most pesticide laden/cleanest produce
http://www.ewg.org/foodnews/

Environmental Working Group's guide to water safety and home water filters
www.ewg.org/research/ewgs-guide-safe-drinking-water

FDA Web site that logs reported problems with supplements
http://www.fda.gov/Food/DietarySupplements/ReportAdverseEvent/

Food and Drug Administration (FDA) information on gluten and the new gluten-free labeling regulations
http://www.fda.gov/Food/ResourcesForYou/Consumers/ucm367654.htm

GUTRUNNERS, nonprofit group bringing attention to digestive health, with emphasis on exercise
www.gutrunners.com

Humane Farm Animal Care (HFAC) and "Certified Humane Raised and Handled" certification program
www.certifiedhumane.org

The Institute for Functional Medicine
www.functionalmedicine.org

Institute for Responsible Technology
http://www.responsibletechnology.org/

International Scientific Association for Probiotics and Prebiotics
www.isaap.com

Irritable Bowel Syndrome (IBS) self-diagnosis test
http://gi.org/acg-institute/ibs-test/

Izilwane: Voices for Biodiversity: Connecting the Human Animal to the Global Ecosystem
www.izilwane.org

Kripalu Center for Yoga and Health
www.kripalu.org

Monterey Bay Aquarium
www.montereybayaquarium.org

Monterey Bay Aquarium Seafood Watch
www.montereybayaquarium.org/cr/seafoodwatch/web/sfw_iphone.aspx

My Food, My Health
www.myfoodmyhealth.com

National Institutes of Health's Office of Dietary Supplements
http://ods.od.nih.gov/

Natural Medicines Comprehensive Database for natural products, including supplements
naturaldatabase.therapeuticresearch.com

Natural Resources Defense Council (NRDC)
www.nrdc.org/

Non-GMO Shopping Guide
http://nongmoshoppingguide.com/

Non-GMO Shopping Guide (how to avoid buying genetically modified foods), downloadable to your smartphone.
http://www.nongmoshoppingguide.com

Oldways—The Food Issues Think Tank
www.oldwayspt.org

Spectrum Organics cooking guide
http://www.spectrumorganics.com/?id=116

The UltraWellness Center
www.ultrawellnesscenter.com

The University of Maryland's Center for Integrative Medicine on supplements
http://www.compmed.umm.edu/resources_websites.asp

USDA Nutrient Database
www.nal.usda.gov/fnic/foodcomp/search/

WebMD database on natural products and supplements
http://www.webmd.com/vitamins-supplements/default.aspx

Yale Food Addiction Scale
www.yaleruddcenter.org/resources/upload/docs/what/addiction/foodaddictionscale09
  .pdf

INDEX

Note: Page numbers in *italics* refer to illustrations. Page numbers followed by a *t* refer to content in text boxes.